W9-BMQ-246

ALL I CAN HANDLE

I'M NO MOTHER TERESA

*A Life Raising Three Daughters
with Autism*

Kim Stagliano

Foreword by Jenny McCarthy

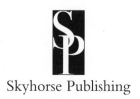

Skyhorse Publishing

Copyright © 2010 by Kim Stagliano
All Rights Reserved. No part of this book may be reproduced in any manner without the express written consent of the publisher, except in the case of brief excerpts in critical reviews or articles. All inquiries should be addressed to Skyhorse Publishing, 307 West 36th Street, 11th Floor, New York, NY 10018.

Skyhorse Publishing books may be purchased in bulk at special discounts for sales promotion, corporate gifts, fund-raising, or educational purposes. Special editions can also be created to specifications. For details, contact the Special Sales Department, Skyhorse Publishing, 307 West 36th Street, 11th Floor, New York, NY 10018 or info@skyhorsepublishing.com.

Skyhorse® and Skyhorse Publishing® are registered trademarks of Skyhorse Publishing, Inc.®, a Delaware corporation.

www.skyhorsepublishing.com
Paperback ISBN: 978-1-61608-459-2
10 9 8 7 6 5 4 3 2 1

Library of Congress Cataloging-in-Publication Data

Stagliano, Kim.
All I can handle-- I'm no Mother Teresa : a life raising three daughters with autism / Kim Stagliano.
p. cm.
ISBN 978-1-61608-069-3 (hardcover : alk. paper)
1. Stagliano, Kim. 2. Autistic children--Family relationships--United States. 3. Mothers of children with disabilities--United States--Biography. 4. Mothers and daughters. I. Title.
RJ506.A9S724 2010
618.92'858820092--dc22
[B]
2010022011

Printed in the United States of America

CONTENTS

ACKNOWLEDGMENTS

My first foray into writing was fiction. Never in a million years did I think I'd write a "Kimoir." But here I am. My biggest thank-you is for my husband Mark, who has stuck by his girls through thick and thin, thinner, and thinnest. Mia, Gianna, and Bella are the joys of my life, and while I'd change their autism if I had a magic wand, I treasure them just as they are. Thank you, girls, for coming into our life.

My family, the Rossis and the Staglianos, helped us survive our ups and downs. My mother-in-law opened her heart and her checkbook when autism and unemployment wiped us out. My mom and dad opened their hearts and their home, allowing us to move in with them when we had to sell our house in Hudson, Ohio. We were like a three-ring circus setting up shop in their living room.

I can't thank my agent, Eric Myers, enough. He took me on as an unknown writer with a single article on Huffington Post as my entire publishing "oeuvre." Susan Senator, a fellow autism mom and writer, encouraged me back when I first began writing and made me realize I had a shot at being published. David Kirby, a journalist and author, read my first attempt at a novel and laughed along with the story, not at me. His vote of confidence convinced me I could make a go of writing.

J. B. Handley handed me my blogging career on a silver platter. Mark Blaxill and Dan Olmsted turned the silver into platinum inviting me to run Age of Autism.

Jenny McCarthy turned the autism world on its head by bravely speaking out on behalf of our children and remaining in the fight long after she could have folded her tent and gone home. I can't thank her enough for the foreword.

My editor, Jennifer McCartney, turned my jumbled-up stream-of-consciousness words into proper prose and did so with the TLC an author needs. For Tony Lyons, Publisher at Skyhorse Publishing and fellow parent of a daughter on the spectrum, a big thank-you for taking a leap of faith and turning "You ought to write a book" into reality.

And finally, to all the autism moms and dads out there, this book is for you, really. We need hope and laughter to get through the day. After all, none of us is Mother Teresa, and Lord knows we have all we can handle.

Kim

FOREWORD

Kim Stagliano is one of my favorite Mother Warriors. She's incredibly funny, and her book gives a bird's-eye view into what it's really like to love and raise kids with autism while dealing with the ups and downs of marriage when her husband loses his job . . . three times! Kim is a loud, vocal advocate (sound familiar?) for prevention, treatment, and care for all people with autism. Let me tell you, it's not easy to make readers laugh while talking about controversial subjects like autism, vaccines, and poop. Imagine if Erma Bombeck and David Sedaris got together and had a baby who grew up to be Kim Stagliano, wife, writer, and mom to three gorgeous girls with autism. Now turn the page and read a book called *All I Can Handle: I'm No Mother Teresa*.

Enjoy!
Jenny McCarthy

INTRODUCTION

Oh, God. Not Another Book About Autism.

George Bernard Shaw once said, "Youth is wasted on the young."

When I agreed to marry Mark, little did I know that I'd shifted my life from Plan A to Plan X (as in X-files) without having the slightest clue of how different my life would be compared to what I then considered normal.

Just as well I couldn't see what was coming when I said *yes* to Mark.

If a light came down from the clouds right now and a voice (imagine James Earl Jones or Morgan Freeman) told you that in twenty years you, a prep school and college graduate, would not own your own home, would have less money in the bank than you did at age twenty-five, would have three children with autism, and would be happier than you ever thought possible, what would you do? Laugh? Cry? Join a start-up religion in Idaho and wait for the mother ship to take you to Alpha Centauri?

Here's the thing. None of us knows what we'll do or how we'll react when life lobs lemons at us like hand grenades.

Mark and I are no exception.

Throughout our marital and parenting travails, we've kept a stiff upper lip. And we've collapsed like a cheap tent. Mostly, we've navigated the middle ground of perseverance and clung to one another for dear life. Even when clinging meant drawing blood. There's been plenty of that. We're both loud, opinionated,

Italian-Irish, and Boston born, and we agree that any argument worth having should be at a decibel level just above "jackhammer" and include words typically reserved for folks on vessels in the open sea.

Our marriage is a mystery to me. And like any good mystery, there were clues and foreshadowing sprinkled about long before the kids and autism came along and the German company fired him by e-mail, and the boat started rocking, then leaking, then listing. I missed most of the clues that telegraphed, "This is kind of unusual, Kim." And the ones I took note of, I quickly ignored. I guess that's human nature.

Or youth.

This book is an "all right already, I hear you!" to my family and friends, colleagues, autism moms and dads, my literary agent, Eric Myers, and some very smart editors, including Jennifer McCartney at Skyhorse, who, like my agent, took a big leap of faith on a mom sitting at her computer in Connecticut. When you finish *All I Can Handle*, I hope you'll have laughed a lot, cried a bit (don't worry, you won't need Prozac to get through the book), and absorbed a visceral feel for what life is like for the tens of thousands of autism families who face the challenges of that diagnosis, now affecting at least one in 110 kids.

My sector of the autism community has taken a real hit in the media recently. We're the crazy folks who are anti-vaccine (so not true), believe in junk science (*buzzzzzzzz*—wrong answer, thanks for playing), and spend our waking hours molding fashionable hats out of Reynolds Wrap. I look horrible in silver—no tinfoil hats for me. Just a lot of questions on why autism rates continue to soar, catapulting entire families into emotional, marital, and financial chaos. The current lifetime cost of raising a child with autism is estimated at $3,200,000 according to a 2006 report from the Harvard School of Public Health.

That's not a nest egg; it's an estate in the Hamptons.

All three of my daughters—Mia (12/15/94), Gianna (7/11/96), and Isabella (9/14/00)—have been diagnosed with autism spectrum disorder. The definition of autism from the National Autism Association is "*. . . a bio-neurological developmental disability that generally appears before the age of three. Autism impacts the normal development of the brain in the areas of social interaction, communication skills, and cognitive function. Individuals with autism typically have difficulties in verbal and non-verbal communication, social interactions, and leisure or play activities. Individuals with autism often suffer from numerous physical ailments, which may include: allergies, asthma, epilepsy, digestive disorders, persistent viral infections, feeding disorders, sensory integration dysfunction, sleeping disorders, and more. Autism is diagnosed four times more often in boys than girls.*"

Given the boy-to-girl ratio, you can see how our family is pretty unique.

If you're not in the autism community, then chances are you or someone close to you has lost a job during the economic crisis of the last several years. Boy, Mark and I know about unemployment, and to call it humiliating and debilitating is an understatement. In short, it can flatten you like a steamroller. After reading about our lives, you're sure to feel better about yourself.

That's promising, isn't it?

WELL, HOW DID
I GET HERE?

Back in the seventies there was a Kodak ad featuring Paul Anka singing, "Times of Your Life."

"Good morning yesterday, you wake up, and time has slipped away."

Kodak moments are meant to be warm and comforting and not moments that make you run for a cocktail. If only life were that simple. Having a child with autism is life changing. When all of your children have autism, that's life *altering*, as if the laws of the universe simply don't apply to you.

★ ★ ★

My girlhood dreams were of the garden-variety sort: I'd go to college, graduate, marry, have three children (boy, girl, girl), and live a charmed life. My dashing husband and I would have plenty of money (that was a given) and we'd take our kids skiing at Killington in Vermont in the winter and swimming in Falmouth on Cape Cod in the summer. The kids would be at the top of their classes in private school. They'd grow up to have straight white teeth and brag-worthy careers. I'd become a mother-in-law and then a grandmom. And when I died, my obit would read, "Damn, she was lucky."

★ ★ ★

"Welcome to US Airways flight 2314 to Cleveland, Ohio. It's a beautiful October day, perfect for flying. Please make sure your luggage fits in the overhead bin."

The older woman in seat 7C smiled at me as I approached, admiring (I imagined) the French manicure and spray of sapphire and diamonds on my left hand. What really caught her eye was the large basket of pink and white roses tied with delicately braided satin ribbon.

"Pretty flowers," she said as I maneuvered the basket in the overhead bin.

"Thank you."

I settled beside her, clicked my seat belt, opened my book, and waited for takeoff. Curiosity got the better of her.

"Were you in a wedding?" she asked.

A bit sheepish, I nodded. "I got married on Saturday. They're my wedding flowers," then I turned back to my book and didn't say another word until we landed.

The meddling matron had looked horrified. Seat 7B was vacant. Where was my new husband?

"Oh honey," she must have thought to herself. "You two don't stand a chance."

★ ★ ★

On October 19, 1991, I married Mark Steven Stagliano in beautiful Hilton Head Island, South Carolina.

Unbeknownst to us when we'd picked the date, Lenox China, where Mark worked, had scheduled their annual sales meeting for October 21 in beautiful (insert eye roll please) Lawrenceville, New Jersey. Uh-oh.

So we got married in a bass-ackward fashion. Instead of taking a honeymoon, we arrived on Hilton Head a week early with our families. Mark golfed with his friends, his dad, the wonderful Mike Stagliano, and his brothers Mike and John. And he golfed. And he golfed. And he golfed.

I tended to wedding details (I'm sorry, Amy, Genny, and Michele, for those monstrous frothy pink bridesmaids' dresses!) and fumed a bit more each day that Mark was spending so much time golfing. We had a blow-out argument about it, which was really about his lack of attention to me, *the bride*, and we each threatened to call off the wedding forty-eight hours before showtime. I suppose we both chalked the argument up to wedding jitters. We kissed and made up, and I refocused on important issues like finding a bridal salon to steam the wrinkles out of my wedding gown.

The best piece of advice I got for my wedding day came from my dear friend and high school roommate, Laurie. She told me to concentrate on Mark's face during the vows. "Look right into his eyes, Kim. You'll be nervous. Make sure you really look at him." Little did I know that she was going through a painful separation at the time, as her husband, a Navy pilot, had decided to spread his wings elsewhere. I'll never forget how she put aside her troubles to come support me at my own wedding.

Thanks to Laurie's advice, I can still see Mark standing there at the altar atop the ugly gold carpeting at Holy Family Catholic Church—thirty-three years old and tall with black hair—the same handsome guy I'd backed into a corner at Champions Sports Bar and Restaurant in Boston's Marriott Copley Place almost two years prior.

On my wedding day, I was twenty-seven years old, standing in an $1,800 House of Bianchi silk shantung Cinderella gown decorated with pink crystals and Alencon lace. My gown came with a pair of lace "modesty sleeves" that pulled up to the short puffy sleeves of the gown. Once my mother explained what they were I dutifully pulled them on, but I happily tore off these "church sleeves" after the ceremony. Remember, this is in 1991, before wedding gowns turned into strapless columns of plain silk that resemble paper towel rolls.

I tried to listen to Father Chappell (I swear that was his name) as we said our vows. As I listened to him speak the words that were going to bind me to Mark for life, here's what I heard:

"For better or for *blah blah blah*. In *whatwasthat?* and in health. For richer or for *somethingorother.*"

Worse? Sickness? Poorer? Hey, Padre, this is my wedding day, and I'll have none of that depressing talk, you hear me?

I'd spent more time concentrating on the limo color (blue not white) and the wedding cake (chocolate cake with raspberry filling) than considering how Mark and I would handle the important details of our life together. "Problems" weren't even a blip on our radar screen, despite our easily ignited tempers, which I chalked up to our Irish/Italian heritage.

Pre-Cana training? The Catholic marriage class did little to break our sense of entitlement to perfection. Why would anything bad happen to us?

On Monday, October 21, Mark flew to his sales meeting in New Jersey. On Tuesday, my family checked out of the house we'd rented for the wedding and I flew home to Ohio *by myself*, toting a large basket of wedding flowers.

★ ★ ★

I'll never forget the look on the face of that woman seated next to me on my flight. I admit that I was a bit kerfuffled at how easily Mark and I separated just days after taking our vows. I'd put on my brave face for the wedding guests. "Of *course* I don't mind. He has to go to work," I chirped as I packed my bags to return to Cleveland alone. I was actually feeling painfully homesick for my home state of Massachusetts, my parents, and my friends, whom I'd known far longer than I'd known my new husband.

★ ★ ★

Even our courtship had been unorthodox.

★ ★ ★

I fell in love with the (first) boy I *thought* I was going to marry in September 1977, my freshman year of high school. I was thirteen years old—younger than my funny, adorable middle daughter, Gianna, who is now a teenager. Back then, parents didn't hold their children back to allow them to mature. I turned fourteen on December 28, 1977, and graduated from high school at age seventeen. By my oldest daughter Mia's age (she's sixteen as of 2010), I'd kissed a boy and I liked it, to paraphrase singer Katy Perry. When I think of what I was doing at their age I lose my breath—my girls are so beautiful, and yet so impaired by their autism. (I hate writing the word "impaired" as much as you probably disliked reading it.)

Autism does hinder their ability to do a lot of typical teenage girl things. They can't go to the mall alone with friends. They've never had a sleepover. They can't sext naked photos of themselves to a boy—wait, score one for autism there. Sometimes you have to find the sunny side of the street in a weird neighborhood.

One cold fall night in October 1989, my relationship with my high school sweetheart came to an end. "David" and I had dated for nine years. I'd fallen in love with him in ninth grade at Noble and Greenough School in Dedham, Massachusetts. I sat behind him in Mr. Sculco's biology class, ogling his golden-blond curls. I was Bella to his Edward long before the *Twilight* series. David was my first true love. And in time, my first, well, *you know*. I had every intention of marrying him after college.

His intentions lay elsewhere—kind of all over Boston, if you get my meaning. Hey, he was a handsome Dartmouth grad with an impish smile and piercing blue eyes who'd been in a relationship forever—I can't blame him for wanting to play the field. I say that *now*—but back then? I was crushed. I'd been practicing writing "Kimberly Ann Kristin Rossi Daub" for close to a decade. A girl doesn't just toss that kind of commitment aside lightly.

Our split was dramatic. Actually, *I* was dramatic (think Marisa Tomei in *My Cousin Vinny*). He was his usual uber-calm Germanic self.

I always yelled.

He never did.

We were destined to fail.

Fast-forward two weeks from the breakup.

My friend Cathy dragged my heartbroken self to a party at Champions. Their restaurants were like T.G.I. Friday's with different ferns and a sports theme. Banners decorated the bar announcing Champions' first anniversary, and beer and liquor promoters were everywhere. One of them was my client from Miller Brewing. (I sold advertising specialties on commission, and I had no money problems—something I can hardly fathom today.)

I also recall talking to a handsome but obnoxious guy named Miles who sold Corona beer and thinking, "Oh my God, I hate being single and all the men in the world are jerks." Then I noticed this tall, great-looking guy watching the Bruins game on a TV mounted up high on the wall.

Physically, he was the anti-Dave, and that's about all I needed.

He wore a gray suit—looking very corporate and adult. Not like a carousing frat boy. Maybe, I thought, he was even *over thirty*. That was my new benchmark for maturity. (Now we get AARP flyers in the mail.)

I took a sip of my Cape Codder and stepped forward toward this guy.

Another sip. Another step.

One more sip, and I've crept up on him like John Belushi scooting across the darkened campus in *Animal House*. I am pleased with my stealthy approach. I am damn nervous.

"What's the score?" I asked, using the female pickup line equivalent of "You come here often?" I was twenty-four years old, and had been on four dates in my life.

Tall guy looked amused and told me the score.

I searched for the next box in my meet-up checklist:

"So, what's your name?"

"Mark Stagliano." (Italian!)

"I'm Kim Rossi," I told him, hoping the vowels in my last name would make up for my bazillion potential inadequacies. I was wearing a conservative, black, knee-length skirt and a long-sleeved blouse buttoned high (there wasn't much to advertise) with lots of colors on it, as if a rainbow had vomited all over me. After the breakup, I was feeling hideously unattractive and undesirable, plus I've *always* been self-conscious that I have more curls in my hair than curves on my figure.

I think he asked me if I was with a liquor company.

"No, I'm not, are you?"

The hockey game progressed on the TV well over my head.

"Yes," he said, eyes darting from my face to the game, "I'm with Seagram."

Now I'm giddy. He has dark hair and is gainfully employed at a Fortune 500 company? Maybe I can do this dating thing after all. The butterflies in my stomach feel kind of good.

Either the game or the event ended, I can't recall. He asked for my number and if he could walk me to my car.

The butterflies are now flapping furiously.

I nodded, hoping my large, blue eyes weren't bugging out of my head like the Cookie Monster at this attention from a new man.

We walked into the Copley Place parking garage toward my car.

"I'll call you," he said, not offering a kiss but just a smile.

"Great," was all I could manage.

For the first time in weeks, I thought about dating someone new instead of my broken heart. As I drove out the Mass Turnpike to my duplex in Newton my Plan A seemed suddenly a possibility again.

The next day at work, my phone rang.

"Hi, Kim, this is Mark Stagliano, we met last night. I'm going to be setting up displays at Marty's Liquors in Newton. Do you want to meet for lunch?"

Ha!

We began dating steadily (dating is what people did before the phrases "hook up" and "friends with benefits" entered the sexual lexicon). That meant we were exclusive, which was the only way I'd ever date. It was a much bigger deal for Mark, though, who, as a thirty-something guy, had played the field until it was nothing but dirt.

Let's face it—Mark was my rebound relationship. Most people don't even remember theirs. I married mine.

We dated for several months, and even went on a vacation together to our future honeymoon/wedding spot on Hilton Head Island, South Carolina. In umpteen years of dating, Dave had never taken me past South Boston, let alone on a real vacation in a hotel. Boy, was I smitten!

Then came our first test. Mark's job was cut in a huge company-wide layoff at Seagram. My dad was an orthodontist. I knew nothing about how cutthroat and unforgiving the corporate world could be to its employees. This was in 1990, perhaps the beginning of the end for company and employee loyalty.

The second test followed fast when Mark told me, "I'm moving back to Cleveland, Ohio. I don't want to live in Boston anymore."

Thud went my heart. How could he leave me?

"It's a quick plane ride away," he explained.

I sniffled and nodded.

Now I was dating an unemployed thirty-two-year-old living in Cleveland, Ohio.

This was definitely not on my Barbie dream house architectural plan.

Mark went from being my rebound guy to the man I cared enough about to visit all the way in Cleveland freaking Ohio.

I liked Ohio. Perhaps I just liked being far, far away from a lifetime of memories with David. Boston was rife with "remember whens," and many of them were painful.

Eleven months after we met, Mark asked me to marry him.

Perhaps you got engaged at the top of the arch in St. Louis or while spinning slowly over the Dallas landscape on the ferris wheel at the State Fair of Texas. I'll bet he presented you with a diamond ring nestled under a vanilla butter cream in a Godiva chocolate box, or had the waiter in your town's fanciest restaurant bring you a special dessert that hid a sparkling surprise.

Me? Not so much. We were at his apartment in Brecksville, Ohio, a suburb just south of Cleveland. We weren't in the living room. We weren't in the kitchen. Or the bathroom, garage, or laundry room.

Capisce?

A girl wonders. *Did he propose to me in the heat of the moment? Does he even remember?*

The next day I asked him, "Did you propose to me last night?"

"Yes."

"Then are we engaged?"

"I guess we are."

And that was that. Hardly the stuff of a Kodak moment.

Lest you think Mark isn't romantic—he did give me a beautiful engagement ring made from an oval diamond with two oval sapphires on either side. It was a traditional Boston three-stone ring. He handed it to me on December 23 at my parents' house while my dad watched the Nazis lose yet again on the History Channel and my mom baked apricot thumbprint cookies for Christmas.

So maybe the presentation of the engagement ring was a bit unorthodox. So was our wedding, as we opted not to marry in Boston, but on Hilton Head at the Catholic Church and a reception at the Port Royal Golf Club. Mark was an avid (that's a euphemism for addicted) golfer, and it's where we'd vacationed while dating. And it meant we could legitimately not invite our huge extended families. We did it to save money.

Mark and I both come from large Irish-Italian families. During our engagement, my folks were still putting my little brother Richard through college at Catholic University in Washington, D.C. We were old enough. It didn't seem right to ask our parents to foot the bill. Instead, we shared expenses.

Our wedding day was intimate and perfect.

I wonder if that woman—on the flight I took holding a basket of roses instead of Mark's hand from Hilton Head to Cleveland, Ohio, on October 22, 1991—remembers me.

The flowers are long dead (and in a box in my basement) but hey, we're still married!

CHINESE FOOD ALWAYS LEAVES ME HUNGRY

Having a child with autism is like a giant game of chess. You need to think several moves ahead to ward off potential problems. "If I park close to the store I only have to walk 500 paces with the three girls, but then I'll be too far from the cart return on the way out, and have to navigate the posse through too many cars to be safe."

I wasn't born with a Ouija board for a brain, able to see accidents, mishaps, and embarrassing moments before they take place. It takes years of practice—painful practice—to become autism savvy enough to be able to go out with any sense of confidence or safety for the girls.

Before I really knew what was going on with my first two daughters, Mia and Gianna, I had an incident that, in hindsight, was where I veered off Suburban Mommy Street and onto the Autism Autobahn. Lenox China had transferred Mark from Ohio to Pennsylvania. We were living in Doylestown in the heart of beautiful Bucks County, and our life was comfortable and secure. I was now thirty-four years old with two pretty girls and a handsome husband who looked dapper as he left for work each morning. My girls had playdates, and I shopped in specialty stores that did not have the word "consignment" in their name.

Since our wedding day in 1991, Mark had traveled extensively. One year he had more than ninety nights logged at the Marriott.

While a lot of moms take a break from cooking when their husbands travel, I always had just enough Italian guilt to make me cook for the girls regardless of how many places I was setting at the table. I rarely gave myself the same proper nutritional attention. I have a perverse relationship with food. I'm by no means anorexic, nor do I binge and purge. I just hate to let other people see me eat. I might enjoy a piece of coffee cake—inside my parked car in the garage—and then throw away the wrapper before entering the house. I'm not quite Harley Jane Kozak's character in my favorite movie of all time (*Parenthood*), who stuffed her face with Hostess baked goods in her closet, but I know I have issues with food. I use food to tell people I love them. I bake and cook all the time. I use food to encourage praise: "How does she do it?" And I withhold food to punish people. "You can have a bowl of cereal tonight, Mark." I'll save the food issues for another book.

So. During one of Mark's trips, I was ravenously hungry come dinnertime and, with no adults around to see me eat it, I wanted Chinese food. I'd fed the girls their dinner. I had money in my pocket and a snazzy hunter-green Grand Caravan (that had displaced my kickass hunter-green Maxima after Gianna's birth) at my disposal. I called in my order to Hong Kong Jack's, which was in the same plaza as my grocery store, bundled the girls into the car, and off we drove into town. My stomach was growling, and I could almost smell the eggrolls.

We pulled into the parking lot next to Genuardi's Supermarket. I picked any old spot. Again, this was pre-autism diagnosis. I got three-year-old Mia out of her built-in booster seat in the middle row of the minivan and then tried to get two-year-old Gianna out of hers. She'd have nothing to do with me. She started screaming a shriek of death, pain, dismemberment—she had these toddler meltdowns regularly. To keep Mia from wandering into traffic while I was struggling with Gianna I wrapped my left leg around her, twisting my body into a bizarre ballet pose. Mia seemed to have no sense of danger (a feature common in people with autism, I was to learn later), but fortunately she only has two speeds: turtle and snail. It's dashed our Special Olympics hopes for sure, but otherwise it's a blessing.

But Gianna was not about to cooperate. I finally got her out of the car seat and set her next to Mia as I went to close the minivan door (this was before all those magic features like doors that close all by themselves, which I firmly believe have brought about the rapid atrophy of my back and shoulder muscles). Gianna threw herself onto the pavement and continued to scream. She had almost no speech at the age of two. Screaming was all the poor kid could do. Most kids her age would have been able to tell their mother, "I want to go home!" or perhaps in Gianna's case, "Get that holy water away from me!" Her behavior was atrocious and overwhelming.

My breathing became rapid, and I felt the blood rush to my face as I approached my own meltdown. I was hungry, and food was just steps away. I didn't own a cell phone, and no one I knew pulled up to rescue me. I wasn't about to ask a stranger to go into the restaurant to pick up my beef with broccoli and steamed rice. We had a neighbor with twins and a sense of entitlement bigger than all get-out—she used to call the Wawa convenience store and tell them to bring a gallon of milk out to her in the parking lot. I wasn't going to emulate her. I was like Hermie the dentist in "Rudolph the Red Nosed Reindeer," *In-dee-pend-dent*. And hungry!

I struggled a bit longer with Gianna. And then I gave up and drove home without my dinner.

Some moms would have left the kids in the car and picked up the food. Not I. I had a strict set of motherhood rules. Never leaving the kids in the car was one of them. (I was also convinced that washing the babies' clothes in anything other than Dreft laundry soap *for babies* would cause leprosy, or worse. My poor mother— she raised three kids quite well, and yet I drove her crazy with all of my rules. Using fabric softener was like pouring gasoline on the clothing in my mind. I was manic about purity and safety from the day they were born. How'd that work out, Kim? Uh-huh.)

The importance of this particular mom-rule was reinforced sometime later, after an incident in our new home of Hudson, Ohio: I pulled into a diagonal slot on Main Street right next to a frog-green Nissan Quest minivan (oh, yes, I remember that automobile). The day was sunnier than usual for the Cleveland area, and dry. I could see a DVD player showing a Disney movie through the window. How I longed for a built-in DVD player in our own minivan for our long trips to New England, or even a sprint across town. More than the movie caught my eye. There was no adult in the front seat. In the back there were two toddlers and a newborn in a car seat. By newborn, I don't mean a three-month-old. I mean, honey, your umbilical cord is showing. They were alone!

I looked around for the mom, assuming she was nearby. Nope. A few minutes ticked by. I was furious. My inner Bobby Brady crossing guard emerged and I flagged down the elderly cop who patrolled the mean streets of Hudson looking for parking violations. "Sir! There's a car here full of children!" He walked over to the car and peeked in. Yes, human life-forms. Unattended. He eyed me suspiciously. In Hudson, Ohio, it was best to mind your own business. There was no Hillary Clinton "it takes a village" talk there.

A harried woman carrying a shopping bag suddenly exited Saywell's—the old-fashioned drugstore with a soda fountain and lunch counter—and approached the Nissan. "Are you the owner of this vehicle, ma'am?" the cop asked. Before she could answer, I ripped into her, "What are you doing leaving your kids in the car? Are you crazy?" The cop turned to me and asked, "Do you want me to arrest you for disorderly conduct?" I held my tongue by some miracle. He asked the mother where she had been. Her answer? Get this: "I went to buy peanut-butter-and-jelly sandwiches for my kids' lunch."

Hello? You can't freaking make a PB&J sandwich at home? You've never heard of a drive-through? Go for the McNuggets at Mickey D's around the corner! This woman left her toddlers and newborn in the car for a good fifteen minutes while she bought sandwiches for their lunch. Ay-yi-yi.

By then I had two kids with autism and a third who was not on the fast track to Harvard. She was an infant who couldn't sit up and had weird twitches that terrified me. My anger at the idiot in the Nissan was real. It wasn't just about her crappy parenting. It was as much about my disgust and jealousy that she could treat her perfectly healthy, typical kids so callously, knowing her toddlers wouldn't try to get out of the car as I knew my Gianna would have. That she had the luxury of jeopardizing them in any way infuriated me, when every day I was losing my mind trying to tend to my three girls, who were so far from neurotypical, despite my rules, my good parenting, my expectations.

As I drove home from the "Saywell's Incident," I thought back to that evening in Doylestown when I left my dinner in the Chinese restaurant and brought the kids home. Should I have left my girls in the car for a few minutes and treated myself to a meal?

Nope. I'll never be that hungry.

WHEN DID YOU
FIRST KNOW?

"When did you and Mark first suspect something was wrong with the girls?"

I hate that question.

I'm a "curebie." That's an autism parent who believes that, in our lifetime, we will be able to bring these kids to a point where they blend in with their peers and can live full, independent lives—through a combination of medical treatment, therapy, schooling, and a rosary that stretches from Connecticut to California. Call it recovery. Call it cure. Call it remission. Call it pasta e fagioli. I don't give a crap what it's called. I'm not going to argue semantics. I just want Mia to be able to live a garden-variety, normal life without needing an adult to keep her safe. (More on that later.) I want a cure for her, damn right. What kind of parent would I be if I didn't? I'm just willing to admit it in public. If people think that means I don't love my kids the way they are, screw them. There. Honest enough?

I know that many things are wrong with Mia, my firstborn. But I loathe ever talking about her as if she were broken. Even though she is broken. It's confusing, isn't it? I write about the trauma and diffi-culty of autism every day, and yet I hate to bring my kids into the conversation. Too bad, Kimmie. Start talking. . . .

I've had more than a decade to think about this stupid question, "When did you first know?" but I've yet to form a good answer. I'll try.

I'll give you the short version of Mia's birth.

We were in our new condo in Brecksville, Ohio, a stone's throw from our apartment. My mom and dad had come to await the baby's birth and stay for Christmas. It was mid-December. I went into labor at home. And my water broke as I stood naked in my bathroom after a shower (God forbid I should have nubbly legs on the delivery table). By the way, it's not really water that comes out when your water breaks. It's a terrifying spray of the fluid that has kept your baby alive for the last nine months. When it gushes, you're about to give birth. Now, first babies usually take their sweet old time coming down the pike. Not Mia. From the minute my water broke, I went into hard labor.

My mom pulled the half-cooked chicken from the oven and grabbed her purse. Mark bundled me into the car. My dad followed in a daze. The hospital was twenty-five minutes from our house. I was having full grinding contractions every two minutes. My seat was soaked with "water." We were like an episode of "I Love Lucy," with my mom trying to comfort me as I batted her hand away, "Don't touch me!"

When we got to the hospital, my obstetrician and the wonderful woman named Karen we'd hired as our doula (they help you get through natural childbirth and act as a translator with the medical staff) arrived, and less than three hours later, Mia Noel Stagliano was born. (I'm crying as I write that. Does everyone cry when they think of the day their children were born?)

Labor made me autistic. I thought about that many years later, as autism vocabulary words like stimming (repetitive movements) and flapping (picture your hands shaking at the wrist over and over) entered my lexicon. I couldn't bear to be touched. I paced the delivery room. And I swear to God, to get rid of the pain, I flapped!

Years later, my physical reaction to that pain convinced me to pursue medical as well as behavioral treatment for my girls, despite the controversy. Maybe they were in pain, too.

Mia was a gorgeous newborn. She nursed well, slept fine, and was an easy baby.

I had no concerns at her two-week checkup.

I had a question at her two-month checkup.

She'd developed a bump on her plump red lip. The pediatrician assured me it was a "nursing blister." I felt proud that she was nursing so heartily.

At her two-month checkup she also began her routine childhood vaccinations.

She was given her hepatitis-B vaccination (along with a bonus 12.5 micrograms of mercury that I never suspected in a trillion years would be in anything given to babies). Hepatitis B is a sexually and/or IV-drug-use-transmitted disease. A mother can pass the disease along during childbirth. If the mother is positive. I am not.

She got five more vaccines during this visit as well: polio, diphtheria, tetanus, pertussis (DTaP), and Haemophilus influenzae type b (Hib).

Pediatricians call them "well visits."

Sometime between her two-month and four-month checkup her head had started to take on the shape of a parallelogram (picture a rectangle with the two sides leaning to the right). At her four-month checkup on April 12, 1995, I asked the doctor about her unusual head shape. One ear also seemed larger than the other and looked oddly placed. Today, I realize that she may have had encephalitis—a swelling of the brain that changed her head shape. Back then I was just another overanxious mom. At this visit Mia also received her next round of vaccines: hep B (more mercury), polio, DTaP, and Hib.

At Mia's six-month checkup we had a substitute pediatrician. I wrote down the doctor's instructions and my response in the blue journal I'd been noting at each pediatric visit since her birth: "Watch vision/coordination on left side to see if preference to right is limiting her. Dr. noticed head immediately!"

Her head was perfectly formed at birth. Still round and lovely at her two-month checkup. Something was "off" at four months.

By six months, the shape of her head had alarmed her doctor. While I followed the "back to sleep" protocols religiously by keeping Mia on her back when she slept, the skull change was not affecting the back of her head—so we didn't discuss this as a possible cause. (I even had that special "never flip over" pillow in her crib so she'd remain on her back at all times.)

I wonder if it occurred to him that she was experiencing brain swelling. I have to believe it did—what else would explain a change in head shape? Why didn't Dr. Substitute order an MRI then and there? Instead Mia got another round of DTaP, hep B, and Hib.

I thought I'd done everything right, dammit. I gained *under* thirty pounds during my pregnancy. I had natural childbirth. I had a Peg Perego Roma stroller. I nursed. I bought organic baby food. I vaccinated Mia without question. I read all the baby books and followed them to the letter:

Dr. T. Berry Brazelton? Check.

Dr. Spock? Check.

Penelope Ann Leach (remember her)? Check.

What to Expect When You're Expecting? Check.

I drove my poor mother insane instructing her on the "right" way to take care of an infant. Bless her for holding her tongue and still offering me good advice like, "Never wake a sleeping baby."

I had a $700 Bellini crib, for God's sake!

I was perfect. And so was Mia when she was born.

At her nine-month checkup, I reported that she had developed mysterious flat, uneven spots on her back and torso, as if drawn onto her skin with a Sharpie marker. She didn't get her measles, mumps, and rubella vaccine (MMR) until her fifteen-month checkup. So what were these viral-looking spots and why was my only instruction from the doctor to "alternate Tylenol and Motrin?"

The day after her nine-month checkup, I took her right back to the pediatrician, because suddenly she wasn't sleeping, and she was sobbing in a way I had not heard before, like she was in pain. She was inconsolable (my exact word on my notes to my doctor). She had stopped smiling and had dark circles under her eyes. Oh God, how did I miss the importance of the dark circles? Worse, how did my doctor?

We had started Mia on solid foods at six months. By nine months she was eating wheat biscuits, soft pasta, and yogurt. Dark under-eye circles are a common sign of food allergies—although I knew nothing of this at the time. Is this when her debilitating food intolerance developed?

I left the doctor's office with nagging questions about Mia's health and no answers. This was to become the norm as she descended into her autism.

One week later, we moved from Brecksville, Ohio, to Doylestown, Pennsylvania.

Imagine this: You've just gotten a promotion and a pay raise. (No, really, use your imagination.) Your company needs you to move to another location. They send people called "packers" to your home to wrap all 42,756,938 things you've amassed in newsprint paper and then place them with care into durable cardboard boxes that cost several dollars each. Your fine china and crystal? Lovingly wrapped and safely boxed. Your clothing and curtains and pillows and towels? Bing, bang, boom, box, seal, stack. Snotty tissues and tampon wrappers in the wastebasket in your bathroom? See you on the other side—you're coming with.

Unfortunately relocation packages are now the mastodon of the corporate world. Long gone.

We settled into a new, four-bedroom Colonial in a young neighborhood, within walking distance to the charming downtown shopping area. (If you've never been to Doylestown, Bucks County, plan a trip. It's an amazing area full of museums, shopping, and antiquing, and it's minutes from the art community of New Hope. It's forty-five minutes from downtown Philly and accessible to New York City, too. It's also near Trenton, home of the fictional Stephanie Plum, so you can pretend you're about to run into Morelli.) Mark drove into New Jersey to Lenox each day. I worked from home for my Cleveland-based sales promotion company and cared for Mia. I joined my first playgroup and relished meeting other young moms. Life was awfully good.

In October 1995, at ten months, Mia said her first words. One morning, she was lying on her changing table (it was a Bellini knockoff, we weren't rich enough to afford the crib *and* the changing dresser) and she said, "Ober." Her favorite doll was Grover, the blue Muppet from *Sesame Street*. Soon after, she said, "Shhhhhhhooooo" as I put on her shoes and socks. From there her vocabulary grew. My nagging fears left over from her nine-month checkup in Ohio had dissipated (not disappeared) in the hubbub of the move. If the doctor wasn't concerned, I supposed I didn't need to worry—too much.

In November, I was walking through Genuardi's when I spied a disheveled elderly woman pushing an empty cart, shuffling up the aisle ahead of me. She looked homeless and thin and hungry. I burst into tears and handed her a twenty-dollar bill. (I was relieved to learn later that she was a "staple" in the store and that she had a home and got three square meals daily, despite her unkempt appearance.)

By the time I got to the fish counter a lightbulb went on in my head. I bought a pregnancy test, ran home, peed on it, and, sure enough, I was pregnant. Mark and I hadn't discussed family planning. We just knew we'd have two children. Or three. Or four—and when they came, they came. Mia was going to be a big sister!

I had another easy pregnancy with natural labor and delivery. I went into Doylestown Hospital at 6:00 pm. Dr. Scott Dineson broke my water with a twelve-inch crochet hook from hell at 6:45 pm. At 8:36 pm, Gianna Marie was born. Dr. Dineson lived four houses up the street from us. Walking past his house got a bit awkward after my delivery as I thought of where his hands (up to his elbows) had been.

I expected nineteen-month-old Mia to have some issues with her new baby sister. She didn't. It was as if the baby didn't exist.

I learned quickly to keep Gianna in a playpen or her swing, because if she was on the floor, Mia was likely to walk right across her tiny body. Not maliciously. Mia did not seem to realize there was another human in the house. I instinctively knew this wasn't normal. Little girls are supposed to love babies, aren't they? It bothered me.

Mia's disregard for Gianna didn't set off alarm bells.

I *can* credit Gianna for bringing out one of Mia's first sentences. "Baby cry."

Perhaps the crying upset Mia more than the average child. I don't know. After her second birthday, her speech became our main concern. Mia had a large vocabulary, but it wasn't developing into sentences. She could recite her alphabet at twenty-three months, and she could also count to twenty. If we asked her to get a specific book, she'd go to the shelf and find it. Her receptive speech seemed intact.

But she used her words as labels only. Even for Mark and me. Cup. Waffle. Book.

Mom.

Mia never called out to me. She cried. She came to get me. But she never used her voice to attract my attention. Another warning sign I missed.

I know all the "learn the signs" say kids with autism don't point. Mia did. She made eye contact with her amazing blue eyes, another thing children with autism "don't do." Her photographs as a toddler show a beaming girl, happy to flirt with the camera. She also used imaginative play.

At our pediatrician's suggestion, she had a hearing test. I guess this was the best he could offer for a child whose speech was clear but not progressing in its proper usage as communication. I dutifully took Mia to The Children's Hospital of Philadelphia (CHOP) and sat in the audiology chamber.

"Mrs. Stagliano," the audiologist said, leading us into the chamber, "Mia will sit in your lap on this stool. On her left is a monkey with cymbals. On her right is a bird that flaps its wings and chirps. When she responds to a sound from either the left or right, the monkey will clap or the bird will flap to reward her for having turned correctly in the direction of the sound. That's how we'll know if she is hearing. We'll use many tones and volumes. Are you ready?"

Did I have a choice?

The door to the chamber closed. Mia and I sat together. Just the two of us in a creepy box with ratty toys waiting to perform their herky-jerky tricks if, and only if, my child passed the tests.

Mia passed. The results were "normal."

I've since grown to hate normal test results. Every test we've ever run has been normal. MRIs, EEGs, genetics. Normal means *we don't know.*

Then we contacted Early Intervention, also known as "EI," for an evaluation. EI is available across the nation. They offer health care and behavioral services for infants from birth to age three who are not developing properly or who have medical conditions such as cerebal palsy or Down syndrome.

A beautiful woman with flowing blond hair came to our house.

"I'm Dawn, and I'm here to test Mia."

Thud went my heart.

Dawn from EI opened her bag and brought out an assortment of developmental toys.

"Can Mia stack blocks?" she asked me.

"Um, no." I answered.

Mia tried. She stacked just two blocks with hand over hand help.

"Does Mia play with dolls?"

"Sometimes!" I chirped, happy to be able to show off Mia's ability.

Mia did not play with the little plastic doll Dawn handed her. Mia only played with her Elmo doll. I didn't tell that to Dawn.

At the end of the session, Mia's so-called "developmental age" was far enough behind her chronological age that she qualified for services. That's how Early Intervention decides who needs help. There's a checklist of what a child should do and by what age. You know the drill: rolling over, sitting up, crawling, walking, talking. Mia was not developing on time, which was no surprise, since I was the one who'd called Early Intervention to start.

When your child qualifies for help, it's a bittersweet moment. You're grateful for the help, trust me. And it's even better to learn that the services from Early Intervention are free. But in my heart, I wanted Mia to blow the doors off the tests and to be able to tell Dawn "good-bye" so we'd never see her again.

Late in the summer of 1997, Mark and I had the opportunity to travel to Charlotte, North Carolina, for a business trip with a side order of golf. Just before our long weekend, we drove to my parents' house in Massachusetts to drop off Mia and Gianna. My sister Michele was visiting from Texas. Her son Colin was four years old. We only saw each other once or twice a year, so this was her first opportunity to spend time with my girls since the previous summer.

As soon as we arrived at the hotel in Charlotte I called my parent's house to check in on the kids. My sister was hysterical. "Mia has autism," she told me. "How could you not know?"

I listened as she stated the obvious:

"She doesn't speak. She doesn't pay attention to Mom or me. She doesn't want to play with Colin."

How dare she! I was immediately angry at her for ruining my vacation and shattering my carefully built wall of denial.

I realize now it took great love and courage and a healthy dose of Rossi anger for her to drop that bomb on me.

Michele was right. I suddenly knew this wasn't a mere speech delay and that Mia wasn't simply a "thoughtful" child who'd rather stare at P. D. Eastman's classic children's book *Go Dog Go* for hours on end than play with another child.

Mia had autism.

Mark went golfing.

I walked to the mall near our hotel.

I went into Barnes & Noble and skimmed through every book I could find about childhood development. I grabbed books by Penelope Leach, T. Berry Brazelton, and Dr. Spock off the shelf. I'd read most of them already, but this time I was looking for information about autism. I came up short. There was next to nothing about speech delay, let alone autism. I was really on my own.

I stumbled back to the hotel. I kept Michele's diagnosis to myself until we got home. We were there for a nice weekend, and I didn't want to ruin it.

When we got home I scheduled an appointment for Mia with a developmental pediatrician at Children's Seashore House, at CHOP.

Her diagnosis was not autism but "global developmental delay." That sounded like a bad day on Continental Airlines, but it didn't sound like autism. Mark and I breathed a sigh of relief.

We next saw a neurologist at St. Christopher's Hospital. His name was Dr. Grover. I took that as a good omen, since Mia loved her Grover doll so much. He ordered genetic testing for Mia and declared her too smart to have autism.

I had no idea what to do. The development pediatrician at CHOP gave me no direction outside Early Intervention, which I'd already started.

It would be two years before I learned of any programs that would be of much use to Mia. She lost two valuable years as we pursued only therapy.

Years later, I discovered that I'd had an incredible resource right in Bucks County: Dr. Harold Buttram, an original Defeat Autism Now!

doctor, was in the very next town. Defeat Autism Now! doctors treat autism biomedically, as opposed to just recommending genetics testing and external therapy. He would have taken one look at the circles under Mia's eyes and known just what to tell me. I am dead certain our lack of medical care and options allowed her autism to progress to the point where she developed seizures. I had only mainstream medical care—but I had no network. I wasn't part of the autism underground. So I didn't know.

He was just nine miles from my house.

One of the suggestions from EI for Mia was that she enroll in a preschool or day care center to be around typically developing peers. Day care is expensive, so that's easier said than done. I was working from home for my Cleveland-based company, which had been sold to a large corporation in the promotions industry. I wasn't working hard enough to make a living on commission with two young children at my ankles. I had to get a "real job."

Even as Mia met with a home speech therapist and occupational therapist (OT) each week, Gianna began to worry us, too. Her speech wasn't developing at all. She had no words at twelve months. Again I called Early Intervention, while looking for a day care center, while looking for a job.

Fortunately, I found a salaried position in my industry with a terrific company.

In Philadelphia.

Fifty miles from my home in Bucks County.

I had no choice but to take the job. The pay was $36,000 a year, a fortune to me and enough money to pay for day care and some new clothes so I could go back to work.

This was my first taste of the sacrifices to come because of the girls' diagnoses. I didn't want to put them into day care. I sure didn't want to commute ninety minutes each way to an office. I *did* like the paycheck. I started back to work in September 1997 when Gianna was fourteen months old and Mia was almost three. Mark was a doll and helped me as much as he could. He was still commuting forty-five minutes each way to New Jersey every day. He traveled overnight extensively, but when he was home, he was a huge help around the house and always a good, hands-on father to the girls.

Ah yes, the girls. While juggling the newness of going back to work and a developmentally delayeded child and the stress of putting two kids into child care, I called Early Intervention for Gianna, too.

I missed the signs in Gianna. Her cheeks were papery and red. Her nose ran constantly. Her eyes were always teary. The pediatrician's answer? A surgical tear duct probe to unblock her tear duct.

She had a hearing test that came back (drumroll please) "normal." All that meant was that she could turn toward the sound in the same pediatric hearing test chamber we'd visited for Mia. She was able to turn to the monkey and the bird to hear all of the sounds. Big whoop. She couldn't speak.

Gianna was *not* prone to ear infections, like so many kids on the spectrum, but she had liquid in her ears at every doctor's visit. That isn't normal! Why hadn't the pediatrician been concerned about this? He'd mention it to me as if he were saying, "The sky is blue." The human ear canal is not supposed to resemble Venice, Italy. Even though Gianna passed her hearing test, the fluid in her ears likely made everything sound as if she were underwater. No wonder she wasn't speaking!

Gianna got surgically implanted ear tubes as a precaution to help her speech.

Her speech still did not develop.

Her behavior was atrocious. She spent much of her day screaming and bolting away from me. Where Mia was compliant and passive, Gianna was defiant and overactive. It never occurred to Mark and me that they could have the same "thing."

By the summer of 1999, both of my girls were in Early Intervention and enrolled in The Community Education Center (CEC) preschool.

I was so exhausted by the commute to Philadelphia that I quit my job and went to work at CEC.

In August, we made what I now think was a big mistake. Mark had voluntarily left Lenox before a reorganization, and he was hired by American Greetings (the greeting card people) back in Cleveland, Ohio. Unbeknownst to me, Cleveland was behind the East Coast when it came to developmental delay treatment and education. We enrolled the girls in a developmental preschool within the public school system. The teachers were kind and dedicated, but there wasn't a rigorous autism program. And while they hadn't been formally diagnosed, we were all operating under the assumption that Mia and Gianna each had some form of autistic spectrum disorder.

Those six years in Hudson, Ohio (our suburb outside Cleveland), were the toughest of my life. They began in 1999 with a trip to University Hospitals of Cleveland, where Mia and Gianna were formally diagnosed with autism. They ended in 2005 with us having to sell our home because Mark had been out of work for almost two years.

SEX TIME!

Most folks will tell you that kids put a damper on a couple's sex life. The sleep deprivation, little ears across the hall, and life's daily vagaries can all hinder one's natural impulse to have some fun in the sack.

Add autism to the mix. Then splash on a goodly dose of unemployment and the financial stresses that follow.

Are you picturing a long-sleeved, high-necked, flannel nightgown *under* a Snuggie? A magnum of Viagra?

I thought about this chapter for a long time. Should I write it? My priest is going to read this book. So are my parents and someday, my kids, I hope.

Mark and I have three children—it took quite a few more tries than three to produce them. We practiced for years, carefully preparing.

I can write this chapter. I can. Here I go. Okay. Turn the page.

HOWARD STERN
EVERY DAY

Mark and i like to joke that, in many ways, he and i have reversed our X and Y chromosomes. For an Italian-Irish guy, Mark is enlightened, and almost always eager to pitch in and get a job done no matter whose "role" it is. This fluidity has served us well over the years in terms of who brings in the bacon, cares for the kids, cooks, cleans, and manages the ins and outs of a marriage and family. Some of his willingness to take on new jobs in the house was the result of being laid off from work. It's hard to say you won't clean a bathroom when you've been on unemployment for several months, unless you want your wife to stick the Scrubbing Bubbles up your backside. Know what I mean?

When I tell friends that Mark does his own laundry and can cook as well as I can (although he can't touch my baking, ha!), they usually respond with, "Oh, you've trained him well!" Not quite. He's a man, not a seal. He was thirty-three years old when he got married and hadn't had a mommy to fold his panties for over a decade. He's picky and likes his clothing and personal grooming to be just so. Go out with Mark and you never have to worry if he's dressed like a reject from a *Star Wars* convention. He always looks like he stepped out of *GQ*.

Mark is the better shopper by far. Back when we had money, he could walk into Nordstrom and, an hour later, emerge with several matching outfits, enough skin care products to care for half of Hollywood, and the newest men's fragrance. Me? If you handed me a thousand dollars and turned me loose in a mall, I'd buy a gallon of coffee and a candy bar and then wander around the bookstore, assuming the mall hadn't replaced the bookstore with another nail salon. At the end of the day I'd hand you $973.45 change and hope never to return.

Mark has a hair stylist he sees every four to six weeks like clockwork. She trims his hair, and they kibbitz about life. He loves going to see Penny. I started cutting my own hair several years ago when Mark was first out of work. After years of bad haircuts costing anywhere from $25 at Best Cuts to $125 at fancy salons, I realized my hair rarely looked any different, regardless of cut price. Every stylist cut my hair into a triangle, even when I pantomimed "not this shape," gesturing a pyramid from the top of my head to my shoulders. I'd leave the salon a good deal poorer and looking like Pythagoras' sister Isoceles.

I read somewhere that if you put your hair in a high ponytail on the top of your head, and cut across the top, when you took the hair down, you'd have a Jane Fonda shag cut. I tried it when we were down to our last month of savings. Lo and behold, because my hair is curly and forgiving, the cut didn't look half bad. Of course, it didn't look half good, either. Color? I don't have a lot of gray hair yet—no idea why—but I have a bottle of Nice 'N Lazy in my bathroom ready to go when the time comes. I'll probably look like I dumped a bottle of shoe polish on my head, but I'll be content to have spent only seven dollars.

Given the girls' situation, I'm blessed that Mark is so willing and able to bend his gender. Find me another man who can tell the front from the back of his daughters' extra-absorbency, Stealth bomber–winged, skateboard-sized maxi-pad. Mark can fly into CVS to pick up his Old Spice deodorant, contact lens solution, and a pack of Poise pee pads without ruffling a single (well-coiffed) hair on his head. All while working, looking for work, or most recently, creating his own company to support us.

He makes a damn good wife, which makes him an incredible husband.

One area where our gender swapping has caused a divide is our broadcast listening habits. Mark likes politics, and I like Howard Stern.

I first heard Howard Stern in 1993, when he was a newcomer to WNCX radio in Cleveland, Ohio. Mark? He'd sooner listen to a broadcast from the labor and delivery department at Bridgeport Hospital.

Mark was a Don Imus listener before Imus left MSNBC and went to that rural channel no one outside the Corn Belt had heard of. Recently Imus joined Fox Business, and Mark tunes in when a guest is interesting, or he watches *Morning Joe* on MSNBC. Mostly he listens to his iPod, which at last count had more than 8,000 songs on it.

I became a Don Imus fan when he brought on author David Kirby in 2005, the year *Evidence of Harm* was published. Imus allowed the taboo subject of vaccines and autism to hit the mainstream media. That genie has yet to go back in the bottle, despite the best efforts of the American Academy of Pediatrics, pharma, and several medical shills who are hell-bent on convincing Americans that vaccines are entirely safe, even as myriad other drugs are pulled from the shelves on a regular basis. Don's wife Deirdre is a champion for kids' health, running the Deirdre Imus Center for Pediatric Oncology at Hackensack University Medical Center in New Jersey. Her "Greening the Cleaning" nontoxic cleaning products are taking root across the country in schools, homes, and institutions such as hospitals. Plus, Deirdre is on the board of the National Autism Association and The Coalition for SafeMinds, two groups that are near and dear to my heart.

I still listened to Howard Stern at every opportunity.

There's a strange confluence of pride and shame that makes me feel slightly edgy, as a middle-aged mom who listens to Howard Stern. I shrug my shoulders when I tell people I'm a fan, as if to say,

"What can I tell you? I like him. But even I don't know how I can manage it." Hint: I manage it because my humor level is on the Stern wavelength and I need the release of an easy laugh.

When we lived in Doylestown I had a ninety-minute commute to my office in downtown Philadelphia. I had a cassette tape Walkman (remember those?) and tuned into Howard Stern on WYSP. One day, they ran the now iconic "Cookie Puss" bit, where Fred Norris had bought his mother a Carvel ice cream cake called Cookie Puss for Mother's Day. Cookie Puss is a hideous cake that is supposed to be an outer-space character with a bulbous ice cream cone nose, bulging eyes, and a high-pitched computer-generated voice in the commercials that rivaled Tom Carvel's easily identifiable rasp for its sheer power to annoy.

Fred Norris is a writer and runs the sound effects for the program. He's been with Howard Stern longer than anyone else on the program, dating back to Stern's WCCC radio days in Hartford, Connecticut, in the late 1970s (according to the ever-accurate Wikipedia).

Howard, his longtime cohost Robin Quivers, writer and on-air personality Jackie Martling, and producer Gary Dell'Abate skewered the prickly Fred for several minutes about how cheap he was and what a horrible gift he'd given his mother. Howard changed his voice on his microphone, quickly becoming Cookie Puss and peppering Fred with shaming questions. Once Fudgie the Whale (the traditional Father's Day cake) got into the bit, I lost it and couldn't hold back my laughter. Tears were streaming down my face as I sat on the train.

Listening to Howard Stern reminded me of our Cleveland days, before the girls were born, when I was financially secure and had no children to fill my mind with worry.

Maybe that's why I've stuck with him all these years. Howard Stern makes me feel free.

On December 16, 2005, Stern made his last broadcast from terrestrial radio. I sat in my Catholic sports car (the ubiquitous Dodge Grand Caravan) in the parking lot of the Stop & Shop in Mansfield, Massachusetts, and listened until I was late picking up Isabella at preschool. It felt like being part of a club. "We" were leaving the confines of the radio dial with all of the rules and regulations and the FCC crackdowns. "We" were rebels and iconoclasts sticking our fists in the air and snubbing the mainstream.

In many ways, that's exactly how I feel inside the autism world. Our family doesn't belong among the neurotypical. And with the financial hits we've taken, we don't fit into traditional suburbia any longer, either. We barely belong in our own families. Autism has pushed us into a topsy-turvy world where nothing is as we expected it to be—or how we would have chosen for ourselves or our kids.

Howard Stern symbolizes being an outcast for me. And yet, he makes me feel like I'm in on the joke and somehow a little better than the people who slam him. If they don't get the humor, clearly there's something wrong with them, not with me.

About a year into his contract with Sirius, Stern got his old tapes from CBS after a legal battle, and was able to replay his most famous bits. On Friday, September 6, 2006, they aired a special called, "Howard Stern's Top Ten Moments Hosted by Donald Trump." I immediately thought of Cookie Puss and longed to hear it again, to bring back that memory of such laughter.

I had my Sirius radio in my kitchen on the fridge in the dingy, yellow house on Reservoir Avenue. I should point out that I didn't listen if the kids were around. Well, sometimes I did, but I kept the volume pretty low.

Do you know why?

My kids have autism. Autism equals echolalia. I did not want Mia or Gianna to echo Howard Stern, since they might say a lot more than the funny name given to producer Gary Dell'Abate that has become a Howard Stern catchphrase, "Bababooey!" Nor did I want Bella's first words to be, "Are those real or implants?"

I listened to as much as I could of the Top Ten Moments throughout the weekend, hoping to hear Cookie Puss. When it wasn't number two my hopes soared. Sure enough, the number one bit was Cookie Puss, and it was just as funny as I'd recalled. I found myself lying in the middle of my kitchen floor with the tears again streaming down my face. God, it feels good to laugh that hard.

I e-mailed the show to tell them how much I appreciated the bit. "I'm a mom with three kids with autism and I was on my floor with tears . . ." Fred Norris himself read that e-mail on air. And he said, "Wow. Three kids with autism." I was really touched.

I've always said that I harbored a fifteen-year-old boy somewhere in my brain. I like fart jokes and raunchy humor and quick wit. Howard Stern delivers them all on a silver plate, along with rapid-fire topical humor and a clubhouse camaraderie.

Sure, there are times when I dislike his guests or topic. I can change the dial when he brings on porn stars who've had sex with garden tools. ("Hoe hoes?") I will always click over to the "Siriusly Sinatra" channel when he goes into any "retard" bit.

But when he and his crew are "on," there's no one faster, funnier, or more engaging.

Our minivan has Sirius in it.

If you see a woman in a minivan with a really bad haircut laughing hysterically while at the stoplight, roll down your window and holler, "Bababooey!"

It's probably me.

ALWAYS ON OUR TOES

Autism has a way of keeping you on your toes, much like hot coals or ballet shoes permanently sewn onto your feet. While most people are working *for* the weekend, Mark and I are working *through* the weekend. We live *en pointe* and *en garde* in order to keep the kids happy, healthy, and safe.

It's not as easy to outthink a child with autism as you'd excpect.

Fourth of July, 2000, we were invited to a cookout at our neighbor's house. We'd lived in Ohio for just under a year, and I was seven months pregnant with Isabella, which made me only marginally nimble. The neighbors Janet and Dennis were also new-comers to the Cleveland area. Better yet, Janet was from Massachusetts, and Dennis was from New York, so we had a lot of East Coast expe-riences in common. I'd never been completely comfortable in the Midwest. The second move to Cleveland did little to ease my sense of being an outsider. Bringing two children who were in special ed only isolated me even more, at least in my mind. Fortunately, Janet and Dennis were funny and easygoing and took Mia and Gianna's unusual behavior in stride, which was a real blessing. In fact, all of our neighbors were terrifically patient and kind to the girls. Not everyone is charmed by "quirky" kids, trust me.

We'd moved into the sort of homogenous neighborhood that has sprung up on former farms from Connecticut to California where two or three builders put up 300 houses using small variations to create a semblence of nonconformity: using a mansard versus hip roof, dormer windows versus bay windows, and varying exterior paint colors. I called it a Stepford neighborhood. Our homes were spacious, well appointed, and a steal compared to housing prices back East.

Janet and Dennis's house was almost identical to ours inside. Mia and Gianna were at ease there because of its familiarity. Unfortunately, so were Mark and I.

We had not perfected the divide-and-conquer life we now lead. There was an "I" in team, as in Mark saying, "I didn't think of that." That's a nice-ish way of saying he was still living in male la-la land and didn't tend to the kids unless I wrote down instructions on a Post-it and slapped it onto his forehead.

While at the cookout my radar pinged that all my kids weren't in sight. I saw Mia sitting on the floor holding her Grover monster doll. I scanned the kitchen and family room like the *Finding Nemo* Aqua-Scum machine scanned the fish tank for algae. Uh-oh.

No Gianna.

I strode into the foyer.

No Gianna!

I checked the bathroom.

No Gianna!!

I asked our hostess, Janet, if I could look upstairs.

No Gianna!!!

I ran into the yard.

No Gianna!!!!

The baby in my belly thinks I've just snorted a thick ribbon of cocaine as my heart rate rises.

"Mark! I can't find Gianna!" I yelled to him and our friends. "Help me find her!"

Now the entire party is headed into the street hollering, "Gianna! Where are you?"

I felt like an idiot. A big, fat, pregnant idiot.

The role of the bad mother who has lost her child in plain sight will now be played by Kim Stagliano. She was born to play this part.

I knew Gianna wouldn't answer us, but there was a chance she'd come running up the street in her little pink stretch pants, blond curls bobbing up and down.

No Gianna. We fanned out up and down the street, still calling her name.

Finally, I heard, "Excuse me! Is this your child?"

I looked up and saw a stranger holding my three-year-old's hand, walking toward us.

Gianna!

Whomp! My heart rate took one last leap and then slowed down as the moment of panic had passed. The baby in my belly wonders when the roller coaster ride will end.

I took Gianna's hand, willing myself not to squeeze it to death, and said to this neighbor I'd never met, "Thank you so much. Where was she?"

I'd have been happier not knowing the answer.

"Our front door was open. She was jumping on the bed in our guest room." I assumed her guest room was the small bedroom in the front of the house. In our house, that was Gianna's room. Of course Gianna went straight to it.

Mortified, I apologized. "Gianna has autism, and she tends to bolt. We didn't see her leave the house. Thank you."

"Oh, *I'm* sorry," was her response.

That was one of the many times someone has apologized to me for the girls' autism. I hated it then. I hate it today. I know she meant well though, and I was grateful she wasn't screaming at me. She handled the intrusion with grace, thank goodness.

With that, I slunk back to the Independence Day party feeling anything but festive, or independent. There's nothing like the thought that your child is dead to deflate your mood.

BELLA'S BIRTHDAY BLUES

I'm no OctoMom, although Mark and I would have liked to have four or even five children. Just not all at once. I think I'd have been a really good regular mom. A cross between Carol Brady and Roseanne. I guess I'll never know.

Mia and Gianna were diagnosed with autism in November 1999. In December, we took them to a neurodevelopmental consultant in Massachusetts named Sarge Goodchild. As a child, Sarge was severely impaired with seizures and developmental delays. His parents were told to institutionalize him. His mom refused and worked an intense home-based program based on "patterning," which are movements that simulate a baby crawling on the floor, and ultimately recovered her son, who went into the same business of helping neurodevelopmentally injured clients. He now runs Active Healing on the North Shore in Massachusetts, and I'm honored to be on his board.

Mark and I had a long talk with Sarge about the prospect of having another child. We wanted another baby. But with two girls recently diagnosed with autism and just learning how much work we were going to have to do to help them, was it wise to bring a third child into the family?

I knew in my heart I wasn't finished having children after Gianna was born. There was another StagBaby out there, waiting to join our family. *After* Bella was born? Hell, I'd have shoved Play-Doh into my tubes right then and there in the delivery room. I waited three months and then closed the factory for good. I knew without a doubt I was *d-o-n-e*.

★ ★ ★

Mark was more pragmatic. He thought having a third child would mean we'd have someone who could help Mia and Gianna throughout their lives. Talk about a heavy burden. I never liked the idea that if we had a typical child, he or she would assume the yoke of caregiver. I'm sure Mark also wanted a son. So did I. Anthony Augustus Stagliano needed to come home to us. That was my name choice. Mark spent my eventual pregnancy talking about Rocco.

Hey, I'm a proud *paisana,* but Rocco Stagliano?

I had discussed a third child with our pediatrician, who recommended genetic counseling. So, of course, we went to genetic counseling. What a waste of time. For the hundreds of millions of dollars spent on autism research, geneticists had no solid evidence as to whether another baby would be likely to have autism. Geneticists don't ask about our family history of allergies, metal burden, immune dysfunction, diet, environment. Nothing. After much thought, Mark and I agreed that a third baby wasn't a smart idea. No Anthony. No Rocco. No more babies.

I blame our neighbors for what happened next.

Joe and Kim lived right next to us. They were a fun couple, with two boys Mia and Gianna's age. We got along very well and enjoyed their company. They had a New Year's Eve party. We reveled. We partied like it was 1999. (It was December 31, 1999.) We stumbled home just a little bit drunk and ushered in the new millennium. Nine months later we welcomed Isabella Michelle to the family. So much for rethinking that third child!

The kids' birthdays are bittersweet as the number of candles on their cakes grows faster than their developmental age. As I'm writing this, it's Bella's ninth birthday.

Some years I'm happy as can be when the birthdays arrive—like when Gianna turned five and we had a big party in the backyard with a rented inflatable moon bounce just like you see at carnivals and a homemade cake so carefully decorated that it *looked* store-bought—I pulled out all the stops that year. Unfortunately, Mia had seizures all day, so our joy was tempered with tending to a very sick child on the sofa while the party proceeded in the backyard. That's still one of our best birthdays, despite the seizures—which gives you an idea of the quality of birthdays around here.

Mia's fourth birthday, on December 15, 1998, was also one of our best ever—at least in terms of being the most "typical" and likely to impress other moms. You don't think there's birthday competition among moms? Of course there is, don't be silly. Store-bought cakes may be impressive, but homemade cakes score points for "love." Home-based parties are old-fashioned and retro, but can they compare to two hours at the local gymnastics school where Lexi and Lulu get to show off their impressive tumbling skills?

In 1998, the gap between Mia and her three-year-old peers wasn't very large yet.

When Mia and Gianna were toddlers, Mark and I were at the top of our game. Mark was still at Lenox, which paid for most of our health insurance, and we had a low deductible. We had a company car—an old perk most people barely remember today. There were sales contests and trips where you could bring along the wife and all sorts of corporate goodies to savor. Plus we got gorgeous Lenox China at cost.

Those were the days.

Our 401(k) was growing nicely and Lenox matched our contribution. Can you even imagine such largesse in this world? We were able to contribute the maximum amount every year and pay our bills. We had extra money! Hang on, I have to screw my head back on, it's spinning after remembering all those things that made our life easy.

Mia's December birthday meant I could take advantage of the holiday theme. I hired the gentleman who played Santa at the mall to come to our house as a surprise guest. I had all the guests write a

Christmas wish list, and then I corralled them all to the foyer and asked them to sit on the staircase.

"We have a *big* surprise coming."

The kids wiggled and fidgeted with excitement. On cue, the doorbell rang and Santa walked into the house with a "Ho, ho, ho!" The crowd went wild. Each child left the party with a Polaroid (A Polaroid, remember those?) of them sitting on Santa's lap.

Top that, ladies! Stagmom has Santa in the house!

As I said, I'm writing this chapter on Isabella's ninth birthday. I went to bed last night sad. I woke up sad. That feels so wrong on what should be an exciting, happy day. The last day of single digits. (Remember how cool it was to just *think* about turning ten?)

Poor Bella has never had a moment of carefree living. Not even in the womb, where I worried every day about her sisters and her, too. She was born into a tumultuous household, where autism had just taken hold of us, and financial problems were about to turn every part of life inside out. For crying out loud, the poor kid has lived in five houses in nine years, and Dad is not in the military.

At five months she had the ambulance ride alongside Mia as her oldest sister was in the throes of her first of hundreds of seizures. I stroked Mia's head with one hand while nursing Bella in my other arm. The idiots at Akron Children's Hospital asked me why I hadn't left Bella at home. Because she's five months old and she can't reach the fridge?

She's a beautiful girl, Bella. Perhaps our prettiest child—and Mia and Gianna are no slouches in the looks department.

Mark and I have never heard Bella speak a sentence. She's said a few words, and has a couple she can repeat. "Mama." "Bella." "Hello." "More." If you say "hi" to Bella, she will return the greeting. She uses "muh muh muh muh" as if she is speaking. We're working on finding a device she can use to communicate now. First she has to learn how to point her index finger. That's the complexity of autism, friends. You have to teach all the way back to the most basic skills.

Imagine nine years and you've never heard your child speak even a short sentence. It stings.

Happy birthday, Miss Bella Michelle Stagliano. I'd like to wrap up recovery for you, honey. Speech first. I'm still working on it. And I won't give up.

WHAT DOES AUTISM LOOK LIKE?

Mia is our most affected child. If you were to meet her, you'd first notice her great beauty. You would not be surprised to learn she has autism. She speaks in short phrases, mostly to make her needs known. "Can. I. Have. Food. Please." She's content to play alone. You can usually find her at her computer or watching *Sesame Street* or *Blue's Clues.* She turned sixteen in 2010.

Gianna's autism moments are usually like bolts of lightning. They strike and then disappear, like when she wandered away from us at the Fourth of July party.

Mia's heart-stopping autism moment lasted almost four years.

After months on antibiotics for recurrent sinus infections, Mia, at the age of six, looked pale, tired, and thoroughly sick. However, I did not notice this. How? Call it newbornitis. Bella was five months old. I was really tired.

At three o'clock in the morning on February 1st, 2001, I awoke with a start. Had I heard Bella? Nope. The baby monitor was not flashing its red *get out of bed* lights. I went into Mia and Gianna's room. Mia was half awake. Her pillow was soaked with drool. I couldn't seem to rouse her.

The pit in my stomach told me that she'd just had a seizure.

I'd never seen a seizure, but somehow I knew. I also knew that I couldn't handle seizures and a newborn and autism. I told my stomach to bugger off. Then I kissed Mia and went back to bed.

At 11:10 am, Mia and Gianna were in the living room where we'd set up a computer for them to play *Sesame Street* and *Blue's Clues* DVDs. Mia had taken to the computer like a duck to water.

I heard a thump and ran into the room.

Mia had fallen to the floor and was seizing in front of me when I got there. A full grand mal seizure, with eyes rolled back, tongue biting, fists clenched, arms and legs contorted.

I grabbed the phone and dialed 911.

Mark was in Massachusetts, hundreds of miles away, with his dad, who was in a nursing home, dying of cancer.

I didn't know what to do first. I was going to have to go to the hospital. I stayed with Mia until the ambulance came.

While the paramedics attended to Mia, I scooped up Gianna and ran across the street to my neighbor Ruba's house. I didn't know Ruba very well, but she was kind, had two children of her own, and her husband was an OB/Gyn. Somehow that made me feel that she was capable. And I didn't know what else to do. I'd have left Gianna with Freddy Krueger if he'd answered the door. I had to take Mia to the hospital. Ruba took Gianna for me. I bundled up five-month-old Bella and got into the ambulance.

Because we lived between Cleveland and Akron, the ambulance did not take us to University Hospitals in Cleveland where our neurologist was, but instead to Akron Children's Hospital just down Route 8 to the south.

The ambulance ride was a blur, as I suppose they always are. I was scared shitless, to be blunt. Seizures are terrifying to watch, and a foreign, mocking voice in your head tells you that your child is dying in front of your eyes, and there isn't a damn thing you can do about it. Seizures are about a lack of control for the parent as much as the patient. I tried to answer the EMS team's questions.

"Does Mia have low blood sugar?"

"No."

"Does she have a history of seizures?"

"No. But she has autism," I told them.

I should have kept my big fat mouth *shut*. Once I said "autism," the game changed. I didn't know it at the time, but most medical professionals think autism and seizures go together like Hansel and Gretel or peanut butter and jelly. They lose their sense of alarm, their medical training reverts to, "Oh, it's just a kid with autism. They have seizures so it's not so bad."

I didn't learn this ugly fact until much later and by hard experience. I sure wish someone had told me never to mention autism to the response team.

Mia had another seizure in the emergency room. I tried to remain with her as Bella nursed and dozed and cried in my arms. I could barely breathe from the stress. I wanted Mark to be with us, but he was facing his own devastating loss as his dad eked out his final days. Of course I had to call him.

"Mark, it's me. I'm at Akron Children's Hospital with Mia. She had a seizure."

He tried to take in the information. He had a hundred questions, like any good father.

"I have no idea, Mark. She just fell over and starting shaking. It was horrible. Gianna is at Ruba's. Bella is with me here in the hospital. I have no car here and no way to get home and you're on Cape Cod and . . ." I had to stop before I threw up.

"I'm just boarding the plane in Boston, I'll be there as fast as I can."

Several hours later, Mark rushed into the hospital looking to me like Superman, Batman, and Ward Cleaver rolled into one very tired husband. He spent the night with Mia in the hospital while I took Bella home and retrieved Gianna from Ruba's house.

The next day, after what was called a "twenty-four-hour observation," Mia was released, and Mark and I were told to see our neurologist at University Hospitals, Dr. K.

Then we were to "wait and see" if another seizure happened.

On February 28, 2001, at 3:20 in the afternoon, she had another seizure.

I remember this seizure clearly for a couple of reasons. I had implemented a therapy program in our house. It was a combination of occupational therapy and other work that we conducted with the help of volunteers. Lauren, a freshman in high school, had just arrived at our house with her mom Mary to work with the girls when Mia dropped and seized.

Mary drove us to University Hospitals in Cleveland.

Again I called Mark, who was at the office.

It was during this visit that I learned how children with autism fall down a rabbit hole of inadequate medical care because of their diagnosis.

As Mia seized on the exam table, Dr. S., the head of pediatric neurology, tended to her. I begged, "*Why* is she having these seizures?" I was sobbing. And kind of screaming.

His answer was calm, cool, collected, and useless: "She has autism. She has different circuitry."

That was it? Seizures are her destiny because she has autism?

Bullpoop.

Because Mia had more than one episode of seizures, the neurologist recommended medication. As much as I hated the thought of meds, we had no choice. In my ignorance, I allowed them to prescribe an old standby med called Dilantin. Worse, because she didn't swallow pills, they gave her the oral suspension, which I later learned was the less desirable option because it can separate, and its efficacy can become spotty. Sometimes the old drugs are the best. New doesn't always mean better, except when it comes to pharma patents and profits. But Dilantin was a real dinosaur in terms of anti-epileptic drugs and had the lovely side effects of excess hair and gum tissue overgrowth. Terrific, let's just add medication-induced physical deformities to Mia's list of challenges. That's just what a young girl struggling with autism needs, right? Mia's seizures grew stronger and more frequent, despite the medication. She began to slur her words, and her somewhat clumsy gait became even less steady.

Dilantin was an epic fail.

I started doing my homework on seizure treatments. I consulted with an adult neurology resident who was a friend of my brother's from college named Dr. Mike. He was wonderful and gave me a list of tests he'd recommend for Mia, none of which had been ordered in Cleveland or Akron. Finally! I prepared a letter with these suggestions for our neurologist.

I was polite. I knew enough not to be confrontational and say, "Gee, Dr. K, you folks have done jack squat for Mia . How about pretending she's a real, live, human child with potential and not just an 'autistic' and looking at these test options?"

Below is the letter that I sent to Dr. K. at University Hospitals of Cleveland after I scheduled a follow-up appointment to talk about Mia's situation. I've saved it in my computer files all these years, because it upset me so and serves as a reminder of why I work so hard in the autism community.

Here are the topics and my questions that I'd like to discuss on Tuesday as we plan for Mia's care.

1) *My goal is to get Mia off the drugs before 18 months to 2 years.*

2) *I was dissatisfied with Dr. S.'s answer to my question, "Why is this happening?" His response: "Kids with autism have different circuitry."*

3) *Why didn't Mia have a CT and then spinal tap and the MRI during her stay? Because her fever was low to normal? What blood tests were done and with what results?*

4) *I'd like to see a detailed reading of the three EEGs she has had.*

5) *A family friend is a neurologist at UCLA medical center. He recommended the following tests because of her PDD diagnosis and that six is at the end of the spectrum for febrile seizures (as you told me):*

metabolic screening including amino acids, organic acids, lactate, pyruvate, and basic lab work.

6) *I have located a lab in Nevada that does this type of screening with high-quality medical research reporting. They need to work with the attending physician. I will bring their file, which includes "Protocols, detailed explanations, and pricing for testing of Autistic Spectrum Disorder for Children and Adults." The president of the company's daughter has a seizure disorder. He was very helpful to me over the phone in discussing the tests and treatments that helped her. Company is CellMate Wellness Systems.*

7) *How comfortable are you going into this research direction? I also work with Dr. W. in Akron, allergist/immunologist who has helped us with diet/supplement issues.*

8) *Mia was on antibiotics three times since November, plus a thirty-day course of Augmentin started on March 12. 11/12: Cedax, 12/27: Zithromax, 2/28: Omnicef, 3/12: Augmentin. Dr. V. at UCLA indicates that some antibiotics can lower seizure threshold in those with the tendency, especially the penicillins. I have a gnawing feeling that by changing Mia's "gut" with the antibiotics, that I started this process into motion. I know it's not medical or scientific, but it's the only thing different in her life. And it makes me question a yeast connection.*

Dr. K., I can't just put her onto drugs and forget about this for a year and a half. I've worked so hard over the last 18 months to clean up her diet, address food allergies, and provide intense at-home therapy. Her improvement is my fulltime job and I have taken this "stumbling block" called epilepsy quite personally. See you Tuesday at nine o'clock.

★ ★ ★

Her answer when I requested the tests that were *de rigueur* in Los Angeles? "We're not aggressive with autism, Kim." She wasn't even apologetic. It was a simple fact that she, an MD with a PhD on top, was not going to pursue answers for my child. That to me is the antithesis of medicine, science, and simple human curiosity.

That's when I knew beyond a shadow of a doubt that my kids' care was going to fall to me, and me alone.

I kept a seizure log for the first fifteen months, hoping to find a pattern, something, anything to grab hold of to help my child. In the meantime, Bella was moving into toddlerhood with her own set of issues in terms of lack of development. She wasn't crawling, sitting up, or even reaching properly. And Gianna was nowhere near under control. Mark's and my life became a blur of preposterously extreme parenting with the single goal of getting through the day.

According to my seizure log, in 2001 Mia had at least one and up to seven grand mal seizures on 2/1/01, 2/28, 3/22, 4/16, 4/27, 5/18, 6/15, 7/10 (Gianna's fifth birthday party), 7/15, 8/20, 8/27, 9/25, 10/7, three dates torn out of the log, and then in 2002 on 3/20, 4/22, and 5/11.

Poor Mia's body was racked with exhaustion after a seizure. I had no idea what they were doing to her brain, and, frankly, the medical community just clucked its tongue and turned its back on her.

I walked away from neurology and traditional medicine to seek my own answers.

Fast-forward almost four years. Through diet, supplements, intense chiropractic care (we flew in a doctor from Oklahoma City to Cleveland to work with us and we went to her clinic, called Oklahaven), and enough novenas to clog the lines to heaven for a week, Mia had her last seizure on November 25, 2004.

I flip the bird at University Hospitals of Cleveland every time I hear their name. The joy I associated with that hospital as the birthplace of two of my daughters is erased. They refused to care for my sick child because of her autism diagnosis. That's not uncommon. Autism is viewed (promoted even) as untreatable.

Miss Bella's heart stopper wasn't as drawn out as Mia's, but it served as a stark reminder of why I fight to help the girls every day.

In June 2006, we left my parents' house in Massachusetts and moved to Connecticut. It had been close to a year since we'd left Ohio. Our belongings had been in storage. The Bekins moving truck appeared in our driveway and, at long last, I felt like we were going to get back on track. Mark was working in New York. We were together as a family again, after many months of him living in a hotel in New York during the week.

With great joy, I watched our stuff roll off the truck. If you can't afford a new wardrobe, just put a lot of your stuff into storage for ten months and wear the same suitcase full of clothes day in and day out. When the movers bring your five-year-old Lands' End sweaters and Wal-Mart "Faded Glory" jeans into your house, you feel like you just had a shopping spree on Rodeo Drive.

I unpacked, looking forward to Mark's and my first night alone in our own bed in ages. The bed in my mother's house was the noisiest bed ever created. Our sex life in Massachusetts was paralyzed. It was like having sex via telepathy—no one moved.

The kids were thrilled to see their beds, quilts, toys. Bella especially.

While upstairs, I heard the squeak, squeak of a child jumping on the bed. I went into Mia and Gianna's room to admonish whoever was the jumping culprit, just in time to see Bella sail off the bed and onto the floor.

She let out a howl of pain. I grabbed her and checked her eyes, afraid she'd had a concussion. She seemed okay. I knew she was both exhausted after a long day and confused by the new surroundings. I tucked her into bed with a kiss, assuming she'd stop crying and settle herself to sleep.

Nope.

The cries continued. Angry, tired, I went into her room. I sat down and wrapped my arm around her shoulder feeling one, two, *three* elbows!

She'd broken her arm.

I'd just won the world's worst mother award. I put my five-year-old to bed with a broken arm.

Poor Mark was halfway into the shower after a day of unpacking when he heard my wailing.

I didn't know where the nearest hospital was. I had only my Ohio cell phone. Would it reach the local 911? There was a fire station at the end of our street, less than a quarter of a mile away.

I threw on jeans and a T-shirt and together with Mark got Bella, whimpering, into her car seat. He went back into the house to stay with Mia and Bella as I drove down to the fire station, thinking that was faster than calling EMS. But the station was dark. I pounded on the door, sobbing.

"My daughter has broken her arm and I need an ambulance!"

EMS is not located in the fire stations in our town. Just my luck. A young volunteer firefighter called 911.

The ambulance came and took Bella to Bridgeport Hospital, where they set Bella's bones and gave her a splint to hold us until we got to an orthopedic surgeon. I'm forever grateful to Shirley, the EMS technician who took care of Bella as I followed behind in my minivan, wondering why my windshield wipers would not clear my vision.

I don't know about your city or town, but in Bridgeport, Connecticut, the hospital is in a fairly rough section of the city. The city I'd moved next to twelve hours earlier. They released us around one o'clock in the morning.

"Excuse me," I told the nurse who was discharging us. "I raced here in a blind panic following an ambulance. It's one in the morning. I don't know where I parked. I don't know how to get home. I have a forty-pound child with autism and a broken arm to carry. Do you think someone could escort us out please?" (Demanding, aren't I?) They paired me up with a nurse who looked like the last doll in a set of Russian nesting dolls. But she got me to my car.

I called Mark and he talked me home like an air traffic controller.

Bella couldn't tell me her arm was broken. She was five years old.

That was another reminder of why I fight for treatments and improvements in care and will never stop.

I've had a daughter wander into a stranger's home. A daughter whose seizures nearly killed her. And a third who injured herself and could not ask for help.

Ain't autism grand?

A CAREER TAKES ROOT

Three kids with autism and bored? Yes. I missed the sense of achievement and positive reinforcement that work brings. Raising special needs children (any children for that matter) isn't known for providing much in the way of attaboys.

I sat down and began to write a novel.

I'm not sure when I realized I was writing a book, but I know how I got started. A high school classmate had introduced me to a writer and autism mom in Boston named Susan Senator. We began e-mailing back and forth. She was writing a book called *Making Peace with Autism,* and I'd just put a few words on paper for the first time.

I sent my early writing to Susan, and she encouraged me. I'll never forget that. Here was a woman whose column had appeared in the *Washington Post* and who had a real book coming out, and she said my writing was pretty good! I was hooked.

Susan and I have much in common. We each love writing, have a strong sense of family and loyalty, and, as autism moms, know that parenthood can be a miserable slog, despite our love for our kids.

We also have great differences.

I am a member of "Team Curebie." I think autism is treatable, that kids can recover, and that some/much/all of it was caused by an environmental insult to a genetically susceptible brain. Susan is a member of "Team NeuroDiversity." She believes her son's autism was present at birth, that families should take educational and behavioral (traditional) steps to help their children, and teach acceptance. She's a great mom, and I would entrust my daughters to her care without a second thought. And I'd welcome her handsome son Nat into our home in a heartbeat.

Since we are both grown-ups, Susan and I have learned from each other, and we respect our differences. Respect can be hard to come by in much of the autism world, but that's another story. And a rather boring one, at that, so I won't go into it further.

You're welcome.

Susan's kindness got me to screw up my courage and dig into writing. When we moved back to Massachusetts, one of the first things I did was meet Susan in person. She grew up in Fairfield County, Connecticut, and moved to Boston. I grew up in Boston and ended up in Fairfield County, Connecticut. We remain friends and writing colleagues, and I value her input and encouragement still. One morning, after several months of typing before the kids awoke and after they went to bed, I typed the magic words: *the end*. My heart skipped a beat. It was the most amazing feeling.

Not so fast, Stagliano. What I had was a completely unpublishable manuscript.

No one sits down and writes a publishable work of fiction from scratch. Thank God I knew absolutely nothing about publishing when I started, or I'd never have begun.

I joined an online writing community. I read agent blogs and began the querying process, whereby you prostrate yourself in front of literary agents who then send you form rejections that read like "Dear John" letters.

I was having a blast, and I no longer felt adrift.

I wrote a short story and sent it to *The New Yorker*, which is akin to my putting on a football helmet and trying to get a walk-on position on the Ohio State football team. I was having such fun writing, it never occurred to me *not* to submit to *The New Yorker*. Really, it wasn't hubris, just ignorance.

In November 2007, I had my first taste of publishing success. Arianna Huffington had just published her book called *Fearless Voices* and begun a section by the same name on her online site, The Huffington Post. *Hey, I have a fearless voice!* I thought to myself. And I sat down and wrote a post. And HuffPo published it!

Here's "The Fearless Voice of the Autism Mom."

George Bush should have appointed an autism mom to plan out the strategy for the Iraq War. From this I know. I have three beautiful daughters with autism—and have racked up over 243,300 cumulative hours in the autism world. I'm guessing that's more experience than Donald Rumsfeld had in executing wars. Unlike our Secretary of Defense, I knew instinctively, as both mother and general of my own little autism army, that my first job was to keep my troops safe.

The autism mom must plan several moves ahead, just to get through the day. A simple trip to the grocery store requires the preparation of a military invasion. Hiding in every aisle lurks the potential for a meltdown. The lights are too bright and emit a faint buzz, perceptible only to dogs and to kids with autism. The Koala Krisp cereal has been moved from its usual shelf to an endcap, a blatant insult to my children, who have memorized where the cereal is supposed to be, down to the exact aisle, shelf, and section. I shop on high alert, intent on defusing problems before they hit us, zigzagging through the minefield of melons, marshmallows, and meat. One eye on the kids, one eye on the door.

What's the worst part of grocery shopping for an autism mom? The clueless nitwits who assault you out of the blue with "the look." The supermarket snipers. If your own toddler has ever become unruly in a store, you've seen "the look." Women glancing sideways at you, whose nostrils flare as if sniffing a shoeful of manure, forehead furrowed in disdain. Fortunately, my girls might not be able to read your expression, but I can. Believe me, lady, I can. Do you want me to roll up *The New York Times* so you can use it to hit me across my bottom while you say, "Bad mom, very bad mom!"?

Guess what, Mrs. Mother of the Year? I realize that my eleven-year-old daughter is sucking her thumb. That's how she calms herself as she navigates the store with me. Maybe you shove a cigarette into your mouth for the same reason? I don't need a breaking news bulletin to know that my ten-year-old has told me that it's Tuesday eight times in a row in a singsong voice that's just a bit too loud for proper society. And yes, I'm aware that my six-year-old looks a tad awkward in the cart, her legs now so long that if I put her into rollerblades her feet would glide along the floor. God only gave me two hands, and I need both to corral my older girls, so Miss Peanut stays in the cart until I can no longer lift her up and over the handle.

We autism moms learn fast how to plan out every part of our day while leaving ourselves wiggle room for the inevitable glitches that tip the proverbial applecart right over. But the main reason George Bush should have asked an autism mom to help plan out the war in Iraq? We always have an exit strategy.

Published on HuffingtonPost.com, November 1, 2006.

★ ★ ★

By a stroke of fate or luck, our twisted road from being broke and selling our house in Ohio, to my folks' house in Massachusetts, and finally to the run-down rental in Connecticut had put me within striking distance of New York City: the publishing mecca of America.

With Mark's blessing, I scraped together the money to attend the Backspace agent/author seminar, at the time held at the Algonquin Hotel, where Dorothy Parker and the literary illuminati of the 1920s sat at the round table and made history. The seminar boasted a chance to meet several big-name agents, and some I'd never heard of. Of course, I wanted a big name.

The day before the seminar, I got an e-mail from The Huffington Post telling me that my George Bush/Fearless Voice post had been published.

Once at the seminar, I realized that the big-name agents I'd thought I wanted to represent me weren't actually my cup of tea, but there was an agent on the panel who struck me immediately. He was a bit older than the twenty-something hotshots, and reminded me of Clark Gable with his dashing good looks and thin mustache. He was thoughtful, his critique style was helpful, and he felt like a pat of melted butter on a pancake to me.

At one point, each attendee was allowed to line up in front of an agent and make his or her pitch. I marched up to the line in front of Eric Myers clutching my printed Huffington Post piece from the day before as tightly as Charlie Bucket held on to his Golden Ticket to Willy Wonka's factory.

I ferflubbled my way through an introduction; "Hi, my name is Kim Stagliano and I have three kids with autism and I've written a funny murder mystery about autism and look yesterday I was published on The Huffington Post!"

Deeeeeeeep inhale.

I can still remember his words to me, "Oh! We like The Huffington Post. Why don't you send me your first three chapters?"

Jackpot!

Four months and several rewrites later, Eric signed me. Fifteen months later we sold a book. It wasn't my fiction, it was this book.

Few things in my life have turned out the way I'd expected, or even dreamt. And yet, everything seems to turn out A-OK.

IT'S A SMALL WORLD.
BUT A BIG HOTEL

Kim Stagliano, you have 300,000 Marriott points saved up because you and your husband never go anywhere! What are you going to do now? *We're finally dragging the kids to Disney World, even if it kills us!*

Sounds easy enough, doesn't it? Let's take a trip to Disney World with the kids. That all-American vacation. By 2007, we felt like the only family in the country who hadn't made the pilgrimage to Orlando. I knew people who went *every* year. "There's always a new hotel to try!" they'd say, all tan and happy and wearing the latest in mouse couture. Sure, neighbor, rub it in. My older sister had taken her son there at least three times. Not that I was competing with her or anything. My little brother and his partner had been to Disney, and they don't even have kids!

I barely remember my first trip to the Magic Kingdom. I was five years old and my family went to Disneyland in California with my beloved Uncle Eddie, Auntie Ana Mae, and my impossibly grown-up cousins: Eddie (my first crush), Toni (my first idol), and Joanne (sorry Joanne, I just liked you). Most of my memories of that trip are from looking at photographs.

My second trip was when my mom took my brother Richard and me back in 1977. We stayed at the Contemporary Resort, that giant silver and glass hotel that in the seventies really did look contemporary. Today it looks like a prop from *Lost in Space*. We stayed for several days and then rented a car (a Chrysler Cordoba, I can still smell the rich Corinthian leather) and drove to Miami to visit my Auntie Rosie and Uncle Jerry. My mom had no fear when we were kids. She took us everywhere, often without my dad, who was too busy straightening teeth.

In 1979, we re-created that early childhood trip, returning to California with my aunt and uncle. I was fifteen and in high school. My crushes turned from my cousins (thank goodness!) to every California boy who walked within twenty feet of me at Disneyland.

Mark and I spent our honeymoon at Disney World. Well, it wasn't technically a honeymoon. I'm pretty sure an actual honeymoon has to take place immediately following the wedding, right? If you recall, Mark flew to his sales meetings two days after our wedding in Hilton Head, and I returned to Cleveland.

I felt like Mark and I were strong enough as a couple to not *need* a honeymoon. He had a job to do and so I let him do it. That willingness to give up expectations and roll with the punches has served me well.

I wish we'd had a real honeymoon anyway.

Mark won "Rookie of the Year" and then "District Manager of the Year" back to back. He was the first, and probably the only, person at Lenox to achieve that honor. With these honors came a trip—anywhere we wanted. I chose Disney World.

We stayed at the Grand Floridian hotel, where I lived out my Victorian fantasies from the moment I opened my eyes to minute I closed them, safely ensconced in Mark's arms. We didn't have a care in the world. I get teary when I think of that time in my life. Did I ever really have no cares?

My fifth Disney trip came in October 1995. Mark had a conference in Orlando. My parents came to watch Mia, who was ten months old and a dream baby. She was happy, always smiling, and she'd said her first words, "Ober" for her favorite *Sesame Street* pal Grover, and "shoe."

We stayed at The Marriott World Center Resort.

I went to The Magic Kingdom while Mark was working. I had three days to fill, and I'm not a spa-girl. Call me tactile defensive, but I cannot tolerate a massage. I feel supremely uncomfortable with any sort of physical attention from a stranger—even under the guise of pampering. I can manage a manicure, though it's been years since I treated myself to one. Now it seems like a selfish luxury that would take money away from the kids. Autism resets your priorities and your budget whether you like it or not.

So, did I mind going to Disney World all by myself? Are you kidding? Remember, I'm the girl who flew home from her wedding sans husband. If I close my eyes I'm back sitting on Main Street USA, watching the parade go by, munching on a soft chocolate chip cookie. I got to see every attraction I wanted to exactly when I chose. I didn't have to see the stupid Country Bear Jamboree because my little brother wanted to. I could scream as loud as I wanted inside Space Mountain without my older sister laughing at me.

The best part of that trip was the souvenir I brought home though. No, not a Mickey Mouse plush toy or a Donald Duck T-shirt. I left Orlando with the glimmer of Miss Gianna Marie Stagliano in my belly.

Mark and I had talked about taking the girls to Disney for years. Mark would log on to the Disney site, look at the prices for the hotels that interested us (the three closest to the Magic Kingdom), and log off with a sigh. We couldn't afford Disney.

Finally, in 2007, we decided we were ready for the big trip. We were settled into Connecticut. Mark's job was going well enough, but we still couldn't afford a Disney resort, not even the "cheap" ones. Mark had traveled throughout his career. And one of his perks was earning a slew of Marriott points. Since it was virtually impossible for us to go anywhere alone, those points had really added up over the years. We had enough for two rooms at The Marriott World Center! I liked everything about going back there except the getting pregnant part. Not this time.

Mark booked our rooms and flights in May. Then he was finished with the planning until it was time to pack his clothes. He told Gianna about the trip as soon as he booked it. Big mistake. He and Gianna circled the date on the calendar and so began the daily, often hourly countdown to the trip in October, some five months away.

"Yes, Gianna, my love. I know" (gritting teeth) "we're going to Mickey World."

That's when my work began planning the myriad details of the trip. The first thing I did was to invite my mom to join us. We needed another set of hands so we'd have man-to-man coverage. Divide and conquer—that's how we survive. The October date made it the perfect birthday gift (forty-nine again, Mom?) from us to her.

Now I had to think about feeding the kids while away. They don't eat gluten (the protein found in wheat, oats, and rye) or casein (the protein found in dairy). That rules out pretty much every food that comes in a paper bag or on a paper plate. It makes traveling difficult. I knew I could pack a suitcase full of nonperishable snacks. What about those three pesky meals known as breakfast, lunch, and dinner? I consulted with the hotel, and they came through with flying colors. In this world of celiac disease, lactose intolerance, and nut allergies, chefs are well rounded in making all sorts of dishes. Chef Mark was my savior. We e-mailed several times, and he put together a menu for the girls. I was assured we'd have fresh bread each day plus waffles, muffins, and milk-free eggs at any time.

I was also worried about getting separated from the girls in a giant theme park. Mia and Gianna speak pretty well, but they don't often answer questions. Bella can say her name, but that's not enough were she to get lost. I printed up stickers with the each girl's name, our cell phone numbers, and the sentence I hate to type, I HAVE AUTISM. I'd sneak the sticker on the back of their shirts when we left the hotel.

And I made up bio sheets for them with their physical stats and a photo, in case I had to give it to Disney security or, heaven forbid, a police officer.

The departure date approached. It was time for me to pack. Mark travels a lot and he's very organized. I'm lucky to leave my driveway a few times a week. I am the poster child for adult ADHD. I am not organized. Packing is a real problem for me. First off, I start too early. So I'm adding and subtracting clothing for days, and by the time I'm done I have half of what we need and twice as much of nonessentials. Second, I follow the kitchen-sink method of packing. You never know when a cold snap could grip Orlando, after all, so in went the turtlenecks next to the swimsuits. By the time we left, I knew I had everything the girls would need. There was every reason to believe I'd arrive without a single pair of panties for myself, but that's a mother's lot in life. Kids first.

Finally, October 6 arrived! Gianna was thrilled. I was exhausted. Time to load up the car and head to Newark Liberty Airport. This was my third flight with all three girls. I'd flown once from Ohio to Providence alone with the girls when Bella was an infant. Never again. And we flew the same route when my father-in-law died. The stress didn't seem to matter on that trip.

Thanks to Mark's grueling travel schedule, he's a member of most of the airline presidents' clubs. We were able to hunker down in one while we waited for our flight. It was more relaxing than being in the large, noisy terminal. The flight itself was a breeze. The girls were happy and well behaved. I felt triumphant when we landed.

We checked into the magnificent hotel. Bella was in her glory at the sight of a waterfall. Mia was entranced by the glass elevators going up and down. Gianna was awestruck by absolutely everything. Mark and I spied the Starbucks and grinned. Vacation!

Our first glitch was when Gianna realized she didn't have her lovey with her, a mangy plush manatee. "Where's Manatee? Where's

Manatee!?" she asked with mounting panic. I'd packed Bella's blankie. I know we had Manatee when we left Connecticut, but not on the flight. We realized that Manatee was sitting in the minivan a thousand miles away. This was not good. I thought fast. We were in Orlando, home to SeaWorld and a large manatee exhibit. Maybe. . . .

Sure enough, we went for a tour of the hotel, and SeaWorld had a small gift shop that included stuffed manatees very similar to (albeit much cleaner than) Gianna's pal. "Marriott the Manatee" joined our family, and Gianna was assuaged. I was proud of her for accepting a new friend for the week, knowing her "real" Manatee was waiting for her back home.

We planned to alternate what we did each day to avoid overtiring the kids, spending a day by the pool and then a day at a theme park. Day one was a pool day. We awoke, ate breakfast—Chef Mark came through and served a delicious gluten-free breakfast for the girls. He even baked bread and packed a picnic lunch for us. Back in our rooms I was organizing our things in one room, Mark was watching sports news, and my mom was in the adjoining room on the phone calling my brother to thank him for the fruit plate he'd sent to welcome us to our vacation.

Her back was to the door.

Mia slipped out of her room.

And Bella followed her.

I operate like Mad-Eye Moody, the character from the Harry Potter books. His catchphrase is "constant vigilance!" That's what's required to keep the girls safe. You cannot take your eyes off them, even for a moment. As good as my mom is with the kids, she wasn't accustomed to having to keep them in her sight no matter what she was doing. Not her fault. I walked into the next room and saw that Mia and Bella were gone.

I ran out the door. Bella was in the hallway. I shoved her into the room.

"Mark! Check the hallways! I'm going to the lobby!"

My poor mother was crushed with guilt, but I didn't have time to worry about her. My child was missing in a 2,000-room hotel on 200 acres.

I raced up to hotel security near the door. Panting, "She's missing! My daughter is missing! She has autism. You have to find her!" Of course, I forgot my bio sheet I'd prepared for exactly this moment. If the kids were going to get lost it was at Disney World, not our hotel! I was able to give a description of Mia to the guard, who alerted his staff from his earpiece right away. Then I took off to find her myself. I started by the pool. Oh God, the pool! It's amazing how fast your sense of embarrassment disappears when you need help. I shouted to everyone I passed, "I'm looking for my daughter. Her name is Mia. She has autism. She looks a lot like me and is wearing a blue T-shirt." Guests were very kind. Some stood up to start looking.

My panic was turning to fear. I thought about that little girl who disappeared in Portugal. I thought about Adam Walsh and beautiful Polly Klaas. My mind was a blur of bad endings.

I bounded back into the hotel and heard a voice: "We have her! She's here!" And there was my Mia with the security guard. I'd held back most of my tears until that point. What relief. Who found her? Where was she?

Mia had gone exploring. Those elevators were too interesting for her to pass up. And she didn't have the speech to tell Mark and me that she was twelve years old, bored in the hotel room, and wanted to take an excursion. She left our room, found her way to the lobby, and started riding the glass elevators twenty-two stories up and twenty-two stories down. Exactly what I'd done at age five at Disneyland in California, with my sister and cousins. She was counting the floors as she went. If you can believe it, a woman in the elevator had a grandson with autism, and she recognized Mia's mannerisms immediately. Mia's voice is rather flat, and the slight inflections she does have are common to autism, but odd to the untrained ear. This kind grandma guided Mia back to the lobby, where security took over. Carol the travel agent from Missouri, I'll never forget you.

My mom felt terrible. And I struggled to rein in my anger. Constant vigilance is a requirement. There's no room for error with autism. We pulled ourselves together and had an uneventful (autism-wise that is) vacation. No one got lost again. Until we returned home.

The week was exhausting for me. Sure, it was a vacation and a beautiful one at that. But it's hard work to take care of the kids 24/7 in a new place. There was almost no downtime for Mark, my mom, or me. It's not like I could lie by the pool with a piña colada and watch the kids swim. I had to be in the pool with them, even though Mia and Gianna can swim. Meals are hectic whether at home or in a hotel, while I cut up food and wipe faces and grab glasses before they get knocked over.

I didn't even get to ride Space Mountain.

By the time we landed in New Jersey, I was ready to get into my own house, where the kids could do whatever they wanted without my having to stay on top of them. Newark Liberty Airport is gigantic. And confusing. We had to board an elevator up to a tram out to the parking lot. But we weren't certain where to go. Mark asked me to zip up an escalator to make sure we were going in the right direction. That was easier than all six of us traipsing into the elevator with our luggage only to find we were in the wrong location. Off I went. I saw that we were in the right spot. I went down to gather the crew. My head swiveled.

"Where's Mia?"

She'd slipped off again, and neither Mark nor my mom had noticed she wasn't with them.

Getting lost in a luxury hotel where the staff is paid to cater to your every whim is bad. Getting lost in Newark Liberty International

Airport where there's a train within twenty feet of you that whisks you to another terminal is beyond this mother's ability to comprehend. I lost it.

"How the hell did you lose her? *You are useless!*" I was scared to death.

I sent Mark up the elevator to find Mia. I ordered my mom to stay put with Bella and Gianna and took off to find a security guard. This wasn't possible!

Mia's guardian angel was still on duty; Mark found Mia upstairs near the train.

I was shaking with anger when we got to the car.

When Gianna suddenly saw her Manatee waiting for her in the backseat, right where she'd left him, she said one of my all-time favorite lines, "Manatee! You're back!"

All was right in the world for Gianna.

I smiled in spite of myself. My breathing slowed down and my heart stopped racing. I let my anger go. Well, most of it. Mark is a fantastic father. He'd never let anything happen to the girls. My mom is the best grandmother the girls could hope for. In time, I might even forgive myself for not keeping Mia safe.

This is life with autism. Constant vigilance is the order of the day. I rely on family, friends, and total strangers to keep my girls safe and sound. Those guardian angels come in handy, too.

NOW ENTERING THE
AGE OF AUTISM

E-mail Message: March 2007

From: J. B. Handley: "Hi, Kim. Would you call me please? (503) 555–1234."

I stared at the screen. Say what? J. B. Handley, a successful West Coast businessman and co-founder of Generation Rescue, an organization devoted to preventing and curing autism, wants to talk to me, a mom sitting in Connecticut?

My curiosity piqued, I called him. (Trust me, you don't ignore J. B. Handley.) Our conversation went something like this:

J.B.: "Hi, Kim. I'd like to start a news site for the autism treatment community, and I'd like you to design, launch, and run it for me. What do you think?"

Kim: "Me?"

J.B.: "Yes, you. I want three things. One: original content, two: links to news the mainstream media isn't covering, and three: to be indexed by Google News. Talk it over with your husband and let me know."

I hung up and sat down on my bed, stunned. J.B. Handley, the leader of the *autism is treatable* world, had just called to offer me a very cool job.

We were living in one of the most expensive counties in America, and our finances were still tight. I'd looked into becoming a para-professional within the school district. With one child on a middle school schedule and two on an elementary school schedule, I couldn't start at 7:35 am or work until 3:20 pm without one or two of my kids needing child care. Same went for becoming a substitute teacher; the schedule wasn't workable.

J.B.'s call was a lifesaver.

Now, how the heck was I supposed to create a new site for autism with zero computer programming skills, no staff, no journalism experience, and three children with autism zooming around the house?

I had no idea, but I was determined to do it.

I realized quickly that we needed a blog platform, as opposed to a static Web site, so that we could have daily updated content and readers' comments to make the site interactive. I wanted to create a community. Autism can make for a lonely life. I remember how I felt when the girls were first diagnosed and how much I would have loved a place to go to ask questions and learn from other parents. Not to mention how much time and money I could have saved.

On June 18, 2007, I launched "The Rescue Post" with this introduction:

Welcome to The Rescue Post, an interactive site devoted to news, views, and opinions from inside the autism community where you, the reader, can contribute to the conversation. Brought to you by Generation Rescue, we will discuss all aspects of autism, from the perspective that autism is treatable and that the mainstream media rarely provides the full story to the public.

We welcome your comments. We encourage submissions from experts inside the autism community who believe autism is treatable, and that the current media environment does not offer the full story.

We ran 187 posts and garnered just over 500 comments during our first three months in business. Not great, not terrible.

The Rescue Post didn't last long.

I got another call from J.B. in September.

J.B.: "Kim, how would you feel about changing the name of 'The Rescue Post' to 'Age of Autism' and working with Dan Olmsted (OMG. Dan Olmsted, the journalist from United Press International [UPI] I'd just seen on C-Span?) and Mark Blaxill (Are you kidding me? Mark Blaxill, board member for the environmental safety group The Coalition for SafeMinds?)?"

Kim: "Really? Heck yes!"

On November 7, 2007, The Rescue Post became Age of Autism. True to J.B.'s goals, our original content exploded thanks to Dan, Mark, and other well-known names in the autism and journalism world, including David Kirby, author of *Animal Factory* and *The New York Times* best seller *Evidence of Harm*, and Katie Wright, whose parents founded the mega-autism organization called Autism Speaks. And we were indexed on Google News, much to the chagrin of those who'd sooner see us drop dead than continue to publish.

Snap!

We cover the news the mainstream media ignores or butchers or outright distorts. The biggest example is that we include a lot of information about vaccine injury. We take the most criticism for this topic. It seems vaccines have become as much a religion as a science. And according to business reports, they are the cash cow for pharmaceutical companies. There's a reason for that:

I recently met with an attorney following a car accident. We started talking about vaccines and autism. I always tread lightly on the topic with someone I don't know well. But I did ask him, "Did you know there is a special court for vaccine injuries? That a claimant cannot sue for product liability as they can when a crib or even a drug causes injury?"

"I didn't know that," he said.

He didn't know that back in the 1980s, following a scare with the safety of the DPT vaccine, the Carter administration created the

"Vaccine Court" to protect pharmaceutical companies who feared that they would be sued to kingdom come and to ensure that they would continue to produce vaccines for public health. Here's the description from Wikipedia:

Vaccine court is the popular term which refers to the Office of Special Masters of the U.S. Court of Federal Claims, which administers a no-fault system for litigating vaccine injury claims. These claims against vaccine manufacturers cannot normally be filed in state or federal civil courts, but instead must be heard in the Court of Claims, sitting without a jury. The program was established by the 1986 National Childhood Vaccine Injury Act (NCVIA), passed by the United States Congress in response to a threat to the vaccine supply due to a 1980s scare over the DPT vaccine. Despite the belief of most public health officials that claims of side effects were unfounded, large jury awards had been given to some plaintiffs, most DPT vaccine makers had ceased production, and officials feared the loss of herd immunity.

The result of the vaccine court is that it did exactly what every corporation dreams of—it immunized (pardon the pun) the Mercks and Sanofis of the world from product liability.

If a child dies from measles or whooping cough in America, you can bet that every newspaper will run a story on it. But did you know that there have been more than 1,300 legal awards to families whose children were found to have been diagnosed with encephalopathy or seizure disorder? It turns out that the children in many of these cases feature symptoms of autism, "aspects of autism," and even "autism-like symptoms."

On June 29, 2010, *The New York Times,* a newspaper that typically champions the use of vaccines, wrote this about a study linking administration of the MMR and chicken pox inoculation in a vaccine called ProQuad from Merck:

Toddlers who get a vaccine that combines the measles-mumps-rubella and chickenpox immunizations are at twice the usual risk for fevers that lead to convulsions, a new study reports.

The risk for a so-called febrile seizure after any measles vaccination is less than 1 seizure per 1,000 vaccinations; but among children who received the combined vaccine, there is 1 additional seizure for every 2,300 vaccinated, said Dr. Nicola Klein, the study's lead investigator and director of the Kaiser Permanente Vaccine Study Center.

The reactions, which occur a week to 10 days after vaccination, are not life-threatening and usually resolve on their own. The fever-related convulsions can be frightening, but they are brief and not linked to any long-term complications or seizure disorders.

"Frightening" is an understatement. "Usually" resolve on their own doesn't mean "safe." It means sometimes your child has just drawn a lottery ticket to epilepsy.

My Mia's first seizure was called "febrile." How the heck do doctors know if that first convulsion has no impact or is going to become the gateway to an epilepsy diagnosis?

They don't.

★ ★ ★

Of course, none of us wants to see a child die. For crying out loud, that's a no-brainer. Because we report on the thousands of families whose kids have fallen into autism following a vaccine injury, the people at Age of Autism are portrayed as "pro-disease."

Hello? Pro-disease? It's laughable. Wait. I should be honest. There is a small grain of truth to the label. Most of us whose kids have severe autism would take three weeks of scratchy, scabby chicken pox or a month of measles over a lifetime of autism. I just shake my head when the pundits say, "Do you want to die of a vaccine-preventable illness?" It's such an insulting and condescending question.

The "vaccine apologists," as I call them, meaning those for whom vaccines can do no harm, love to holler about "herd immunity." That means that unless a certain percentage of the population is immunized, a disease can spread. That's all well and good in theory. But when it's your little calf who falls, herd immunity doesn't sound too good.

A child born in 2010 will receive forty-eight vaccinations from birth through age six if they follow The Centers for Disease Control (CDC) vaccination schedule. Since a lot of folks won't believe me on that, I'll list them for you.

Birth: hepatitis B

Two months: hepatitis B, rotavirus, diphtheria, tetanus, pertussis, Haemophilus influenza, pneumococcal, polio

Four months: rotavirus, diphtheria, tetanus, pertussis, Haemophilus influenza, pneumococcal, polio

Six months: hepatitis B, rotavirus, diphtheria, tetanus, pertussis, Haemophilus influenza, pneumococcal, seasonal flu

Twelve–fifteen months: diphtheria, tetanus, pertussis, Haemophilus influenza, pneumococcal, polio, measles, mumps, rubella, hepatitis A, chicken pox

Two years: seasonal flu, hepatitis A

Three years: seasonal flu

Four years: seasonal flu, diphtheria, tetanus, pertussis, polio, measles, mumps, rubella, chicken pox

Five years: seasonal flu

The first shot comes on the day a baby is born, when he is inoculated for hepatitis B, which is a disease transmitted sexually or through IV drug use. Not even the craziest rock star's kids are shooting up or having sex in the nursery. There's a Web site called www.iansvoice. org. Ian suffered a rare—but real—allergic reaction to an ingredient in his birth hepatitis B vaccination. He swelled up like a Macy's

Thanksgiving Day parade balloon and the blessed child never recovered. He died at forty-seven days of age.

In the spring of 2010, I received an e-mail from a woman who had just been awarded six figures by the vaccine court because she had been neurologically injured by a common seasonal flu vaccine. She lost four years of her health. Thank God she recovered.

You can get a flu shot in the grocery store every fall and winter, administered by a poorly paid health aide who the month before might have been bagging your groceries for you.

Vaccine safety and informed parental consent is one of our hottest topics at Age of Autism in that it draws the most critics, to which I say, "Bring it on."

It is my great responsibility and honor to sound the alarm bells about the autism epidemic every day. Believe it or not, there are people (some with autism, some just lacking in empathy, others trying to save their own political, professional, and economic arses) who want the general public to think autism has always been with us in these numbers. If so, please look under your bed, chances are there is a gaggle of fifty-year-old autistic men hiding there. Some people claim it's just *better diagnosis* and/or what's called diagnostic substitution, meaning people who would have been called mentally retarded in 1965 are being labeled autistic today. Not even the last loser in the class at Tick Tock Tech Medical School could fail to recognize autism in the children I see every day. It doesn't look like cognitive challenges or Down syndrome. It looks like autism. From *Medical News Today*: "A study by researchers at University of California's Davis M.I.N.D. Institute has found that the seven- to eight-fold increase in the number of children born in California with autism since 1990 cannot be explained by either changes in how the condition is diagnosed or counted—and the trend shows no sign of abating."

I admit to using less precise methods of deduction. I looked at my three kids versus the rest of my family tree for the last three generations. I asked my childhood babysitter, who was a special education teacher in Massachusetts in the early 1970s, how many students with autism she had in her self-contained classroom. "None."

There are bloggers and advocates within the autism community who preach that autism is a set of nifty special traits, like a Swiss Army knife for life. *Oy vey.* The media loves to pick up the odd story about the autistic boy who scored twenty points in the last three minutes of a basketball game. What about the rest of the child's life and his prospects for the future? Do they cover that?

I've spent enough time with high-functioning adults with autism and Asperger's to realize that while the skills their diagnosis might bring in terms of memory, focus, or talents in a specific area—the depression, lack of ability to find and hold a job, difficulty in forming romantic relationships, and sense of detachment from the world can be very painful.

I met a wonderful woman with Asperger's in my town. She worked at the grocery store. She was fired because she couldn't stop talking to customers about certain products they were buying—like pregnancy tests. Not everyone who buys a preggers kit is thrilled with the prospect of pregnancy, and hardly anyone wants to chat about it with the checkout clerk. This gal could not stop asking inappropriate questions, despite requests from her supervisors. I know that she's a warm, giving woman, very smart (working on a graduate degree) and capable.

She lost her job at a grocery store.

Our work at Age of Autism is disliked by many people because we shine a light on the autism crisis. I think that's great. I don't ever want to be a scoop of vanilla ice cream melting in a white bowl of obscurity. What's the point in playing it safe all the time?

I once accused an autism blogger of wearing Kevlar pantyhose because she straddled the fence so consistently, never offering a strong opinion. That's just not my way.

At the end of the day, if we can move awareness beyond the ads featuring bright-eyed, healthy-looking kids with a voice-over saying, "Your child has a better chance of being diagnosed with autism than playing major league baseball" and into the harsher realities of autism, we'll help people at both ends of the spectrum.

Advertising 101: Fear and ugly images sell charity. Sally Struthers didn't hold a plump, well-fed child to encourage donations to Save the Children. Heck, even the dogs and cats in the animal charity ads look forlorn.

Here's my idea for an ad: How about a photo of a bedroom with the walls smeared with poop, mattress on the floor, and a twelve-year-old boy punching holes into the walls as his parents (mom with a bloody lip) try to calm him.

That's autism in a lot of households.

It's not politically correct to mention the dirty, smelly, poopy, angry, screaming, fear-inducing side of autism.

Which is exactly why I make sure we do that on Age of Autism and in my writing on Huffington Post and elsewhere.

In 2009, an eighteen-year-old boy named Sky Walker allegedly beat his mother, Trudy Steuernagel, a professor at Kent State University in Kent, Ohio, to death in their kitchen. He spent months in a jail cell. And he now lives in an institution. I wrote about Sky—his story is a cautionary tale. Little boys with autism grow up into grown men with autism. Sky's mother wrote a letter to her family to be read in the event of her death. She predicted her son would kill her.

Where's the alarm over autism, the escalating numbers, the future?

We just spent six months and billions of dollars panicking the American public about the H1N1 virus. Epidemiologists predicted death on a massive scale, and the pharmaceutical companies whipped out the vaccine version of a microwave cake. People who wouldn't buy a car in its first model year lined up for this shot, complete with twenty-five micrograms of mercury in every dose. Madonn'.

We know how many mistresses Tiger Woods bedded and how much Botox was injected into OctoMom's face. We followed the balloon boy on Twitter and the nightly news (guilty) and lamented the time slot NBC would eventually give Jay Leno, but we can't get experts to wake up and smell the autism epidemic that's churning behind us. The CDC announced the latest increase in autism prevalence, 1 in 150 is now 1 in 110, on the Friday *before Christmas*—the blackest of the media black holes. Friday afternoon is when organizations traditionally release information that they would rather have disappear into the weekend without much media attention.

It seems no one in our government is willing to declare autism an emergency, even though it is an epidemic that continues to grow year after year and is likely to have a huge impact on our Social Security system. Lord, when H1N1 hit our shores, you'd have thought it was raining anthrax and Ebola the way the media hyped up every sneeze and sniffle from Portland to San Diego. But autism on the rise? Crickets chirped.

So at Age of Autism we wrote about the numbers and Tweeted them to death for over two weeks.

David beat Goliath, this I know. For the Bible tells me so.

Age of Autism is our slingshot.

THE AUTISM MARRIAGE: SOUL MATES OR CELL MATES?

"Eighty percent of autism marriages end in divorce." this statement on the difficulty of having an autistic child is bandied about frequently, though I'm not sure there are stats to prove it. As far as I can see, most of my friends who have an autistic child have remained married.

"One hundred percent of autism marriages have an inordinate amount of stress" is pretty much dead-on accurate. I made that stat up myself having lived it for the last fifteen-plus years.

Mark and I never imagined we'd face autism and unemployment and a global economic collapse when we got married. Nostradamus couldn't have predicted the crap we've had to deal with day in and day out.

To the fly on the wall, Mark and I might appear to have a dreadful marriage. We yell a lot. We shake our heads and gesture with our arms like crazy people. We cruise around the house picking up messes, checking to see if bathroom doors are locked, and shuttling yet another load of laundry to the washing machine. I'm on my computer off and on from 6:00 am to 9:00 pm writing and managing Age of Autism. Mark is at his desk writing orders, following up with vendors, and Tweeting his politics. (I love his sense of justice, honed by our difficulties over the years.) We've gone through periods when sex is like Halley's Comet, an infrequent visitor.

Like all married couples, Mark and I share an unspoken language. "Did you . . ." comes out of his mouth, and I know he's going to ask if I took Bella to the bathroom within the hour. I'll say, "Can you . . ." and he empties the trash can or the dishwasher.

We began our marriage as two independent people. We've never been attached at the hip. Now, almost twenty years later, we're a pretty well-oiled machine, and I feel like we're as secure in our marriage as a couple can be. However, that wasn't always the case. If it hadn't been for our Catholic sense of duty to each other, and our kids, we might well have ended up a statistic, too.

When we were first married, and before the kids arrived, Mark had joined a country club in Aurora, Ohio. We had enough money back then for a country club! I'd learned to accept his golf, albeit begrudgingly. Heck, we were married at a golf resort. He did what he wanted and so did I.

During the summer of 2000, I was in my last trimester with Bella. Mia and Gianna were proving to be anything but typical, while Mark was playing the role of a typical, corporate spouse. Circa 1965. I was overwhelmed by the kids, with a gigantic house to clean, and I was pregnant.

My pre-marriage ideal of the company-man husband was back-firing badly. He bragged that he'd played 100 rounds of golf in a single season. In dreary, rainy, cold Cleveland, Ohio, that's quite an achievement. A round of golf took him away from the family for at least five hours, usually seven or eight on weekends. That adds up to approximately thirty days a year spent at the country club instead of with us.

One Saturday afternoon when Mark had been gone for several hours, and I'd been lumbering around the house pregnant, trying to care for two children with autism, five-year-old Mia had an accident in her bedroom. She stepped out of her soiled pants, took the blob of poop in her hands, squished it, dropped it, stepped in it, and then walked up and down the upstairs hallway, with her hands on the walls.

The sight stopped me in my tracks. The walls and carpeting were covered in poop. Mia was filthy, standing in the hallway and looking at me with her big blue eyes. Gianna was traipsing through the poop, oblivious to the mess.

I lost it.

I yelled. I screamed. I sobbed. I didn't know where to begin. The walls? The carpet? The children? The liquor cabinet?

The smell nauseated me. The view made me see red.

I cleaned up as much as I could, and then I sat on the stairs and cried. I was so angry at Mark. Where the hell was he when I needed him? At the goddamned golf course.

Things didn't improve from there. We grew further apart.

Mark left American Greetings and became General Manager for a German housewares company called Leifheit. The new job came with a sizable salary increase. We needed every penny to meet our rising bills. Assuming we kept to a budget.

And what did Mark do?

He cruised into our driveway in a black BMW 330xi.

I tried to hate that car. But, Lord, it was sweet! I *did* hate that Mark didn't tell me he was going to lease it. He'd had a company car at American Greetings and a car allowance with Leifheit. He spent the monthly allowance and then some at BMW.

Like a four-year-old trying to convince his mom why he absolutely had to have that second piece of cake, Mark's explanation for the BMW was that he was now working for a German company, so the German car made sense. To which I answered, "Sure, how about a $25,000 Volkswagen Jetta?"

Fast-forward to a sunny Saturday in July. We awoke to Mia's horrible sucking sounds that signaled a seizure. I knew she was in for a day of grand mal seizures, and that I would have to be at her side. Bella was nine months old. Gianna was five and still pretty nutty.

Being Saturday, Mark had a round of golf lined up. I looked at him like he was crazy as he got up to shower.

"Are you going to the club?"

"I promised Mike I'd play with him. I'll be home early."

How about an early grave? He was going to leave me for the day because of a promise he'd made to his brother about a round of golf!

Bitterness became the flavor of the week.

He went golfing.

Mark's dad had passed away in February 2001, and his mother generously gave each of her children a monetary gift. Mark could plainly see that I was cracking under the stress of the children. His answer? Hire someone to do the work he didn't want to do so that his lifestyle wouldn't have to change. We used the money to pay for autism treatments and to hire live-in help.

In September 2001, we welcomed an au pair from South Africa named Cindy J. into our home. She was a godsend, and we enjoyed having her live with us for almost three years. Our house had a large finished basement so we were able to create a suite for Cindy. Having her around meant I could leave the house alone— joy!

One trip that I was able to make alone wasn't so joyful. Call it my Elin Woods moment without the other woman.

My anger at Mark had been bubbling up since he'd left the hose at 7:00 am to, yes, go golfing. It was 3:30 pm, and he hadn't come home. I don't remember what set me off. I think we had a date planned and he was late. I was consumed with anger and frustration. I told Cindy I was going out, and I raced over to the golf course.

I flounced into the grill room and saw Mark sitting at the bar. I grabbed his arm and said, "Come outside with me right now!" The guys at that bar looked aghast.

We stood in front of the clubhouse, and I announced to Mark, "I spend all of my time with the kids. You're always here. I'm thirty-eight years old, and I AM LONELY! I don't love you any-more, and I want a divorce!"

I was not using my indoor voice.

Mark tried to calm me down. Fat chance. I stomped back to my minivan as he walked toward the pro shop, nothing resolved. I shot out of the parking lot, put down my window, and gave him (and everyone on the practice putting green) the finger.

It wasn't just the golf that ticked me off. Mark had changed. At least I thought he had. When we returned to Ohio, I was no longer working, I had two kids who did not fit into the surburban mold of dancing classes (note, never take a child with noise issues to tap-dancing class) and T-ball and tea parties. My time was spent looking for size-six Pampers for two kids who had no interest in toilet training. I was approaching forty and feeling anything but fabulous.

I pretended everything was fine as we paraded around town in his black BMW listening to the *Sopranos* soundtrack thinking we were a couple of big swinging dicks.

As I look back, everything *was* fine. He was working, we had a lovely house, our three beautiful kids were making progress, and we'd accepted their challenges with purpose and grace. What was I such a bitch about? Golf? He wasn't sexting other women, or gambling, or drinking away his paycheck.

Things could have been much worse.

And so, they got much worse.

Mark and I were in a period of calm and relative happiness. It was autumn of 2003, and the golf season was drawing to a close. Amen! Mark received an invitation to a grand opening for Legacy Village—one of those destination shopping centers that look like they were designed by Walt Disney. Cindy watched the kids; Mark and I hopped into the Beemer and off we went to this invitation-only shopping event.

Oh, we shopped! Mark bought me several outfits at one of the snazzy stores. By snazzy, I mean the sort of store that lets you *keep* the hanger, and might even give you a gift box. It was a lovely night. And the last night of life as we knew it.

The next morning Mark received an e-mail from Germany, firing him from his job with Leifheit.

Just like that, we joined the ranks of the unemployed. Mark was stunned. Sales were up—the products were in prestigious retailers and fancy catalogs.

They never called him. He didn't hear from a soul in Germany again. That day, I drove back to Legacy Village and returned the clothes we'd bought the night before. Everything had changed.

Including Mark and me. Suddenly he saw what our household was really like. He didn't have a job to distract him from the circus we called Chez Stagliano. I realized that golf was the least of my worries.

And so we navigated the new world of unemployment. We didn't expect to get citizenship, though.

A PAPER MITTEN ON
THE GIVING TREE

You haven't lived until you've been a name on a paper mitten on the church giving tree. Twice.

In December 2004, Mark had been out of work for fourteen months. Our severance pay was long gone. We'd ripped through our savings like toilet paper on your first night in Mexico. And Mark's mother had started to support us financially. I call that the Trifecta of Depression.

The year before, the Rossi family (my folks, my sister, her husband and son, my brother and his partner) had come to Hudson, Ohio, to spend the holiday in our idyllic Currier and Ives town. Hudson personifies charming at the holidays—from the brick clock tower with the giant Hickory Dickory Dock mouse running down it, to the New England–style town green festooned with wreaths and lights, to the Main Street that still boasted an old-fashioned drugstore with a soda fountain and lunch counter.

Mark had been out of work since October, but I had no sense of panic, yet. It never occurred to me that Mark wouldn't find another good-paying job quickly. I understood we'd probably have to leave Hudson, but that didn't faze me in the least. I liked Ohio well enough, but it wasn't "home," and I knew the girls could do better elsewhere as far as special education in the schools went.

I secured a three-bedroom bed-and-breakfast for the family in a Victorian house one gingerbread cut from being a cliché. I decked

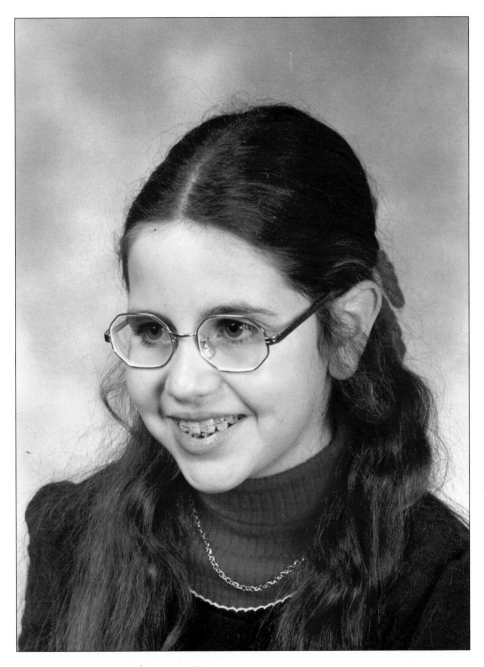

Kim in sixth grade at Dominican Academy

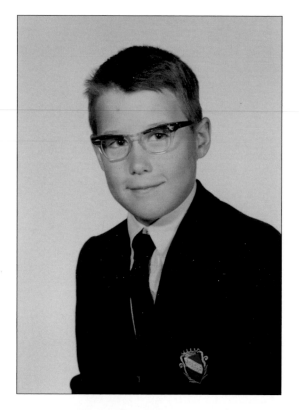

Mark in third grade at St. John the Evangelist, Rochester, NY

Mark and Kim, 1990, Hilton Head, SC

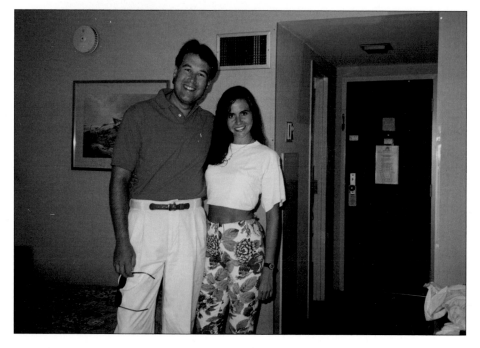

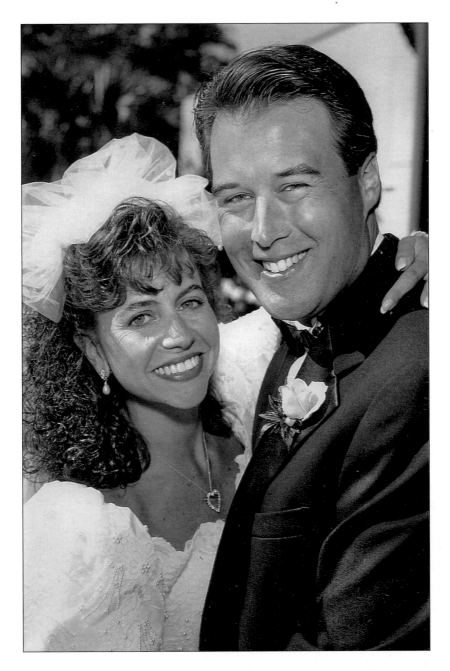

Mark and Kim's wedding day, October 19, 1991, Hilton Head, SC

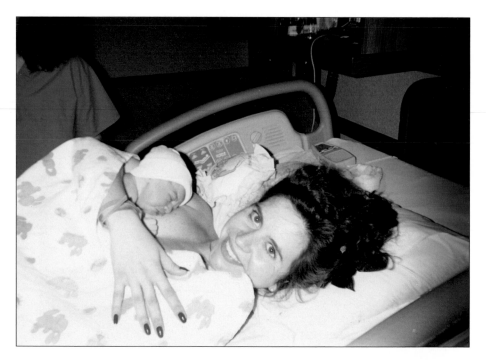

Mia's birth day, December 15, 1994

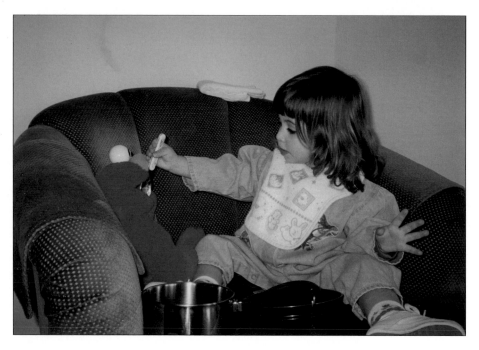

Mia showing off her social play skills before her diagnosis

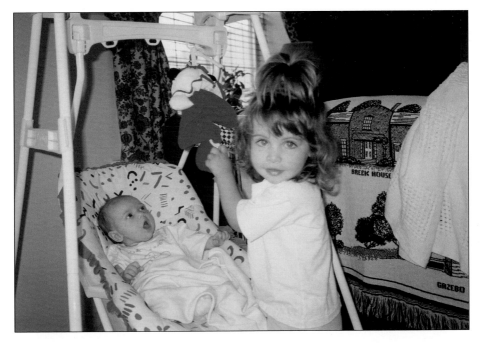

Baby Gianna with Mia

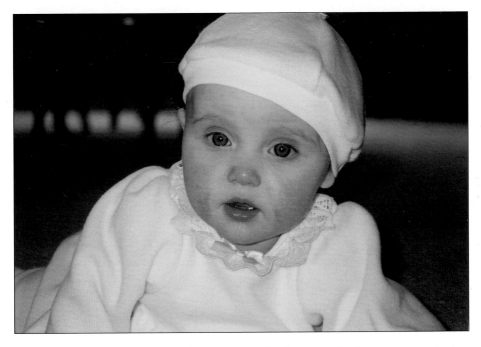

Gianna with rheumy eyes and red, papery cheeks

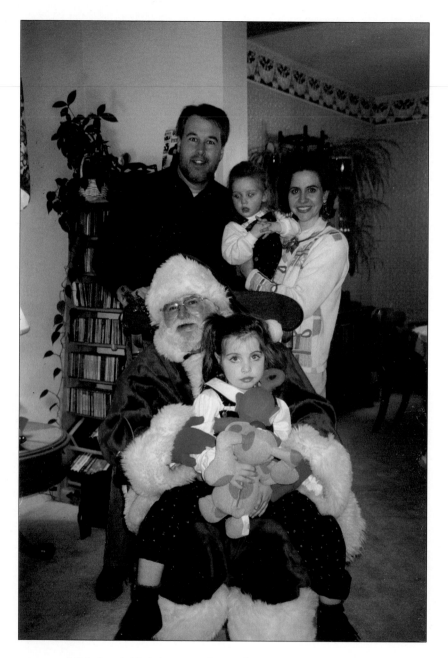

Mia's fourth birthday party, December 1998, Doylestown, PA

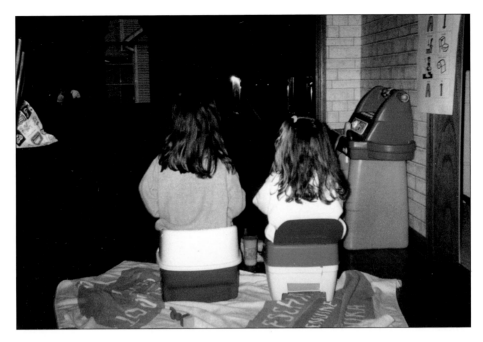

Mia and Gianna potty training

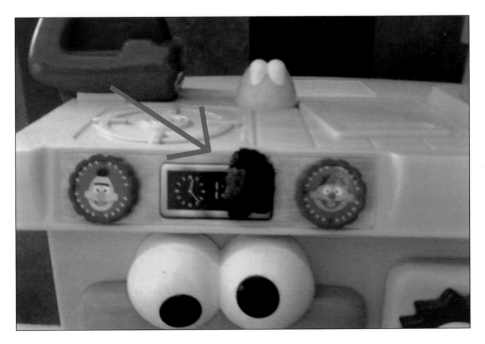

The Sesame Street Kitchen after the famous crapisode. Note the extra button.

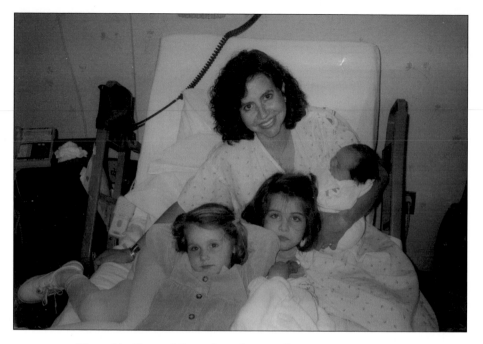

Kim with Gianna, Mia, and newborn Bella, September 15, 2000

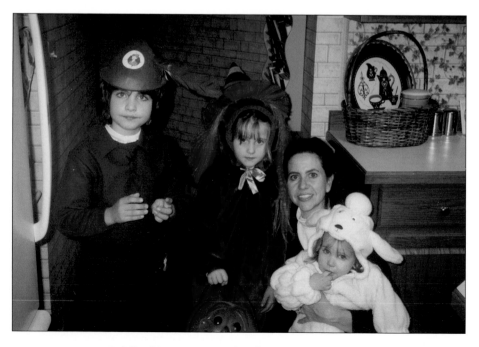

Mia, Gianna, Kim, and Bella, Halloween 2001

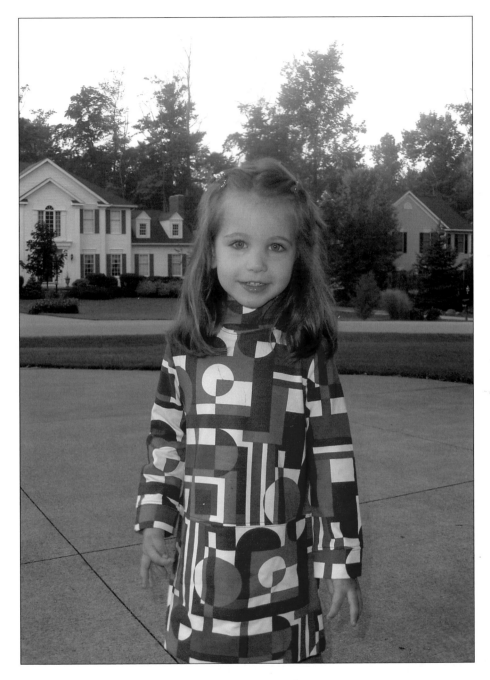

Bella, four years old, Hudson, Ohio, fall 2004

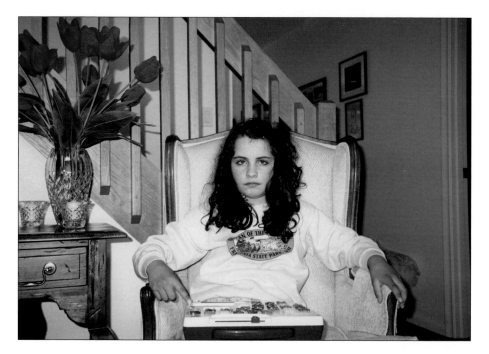

Mia, looking grim before a seizure episode

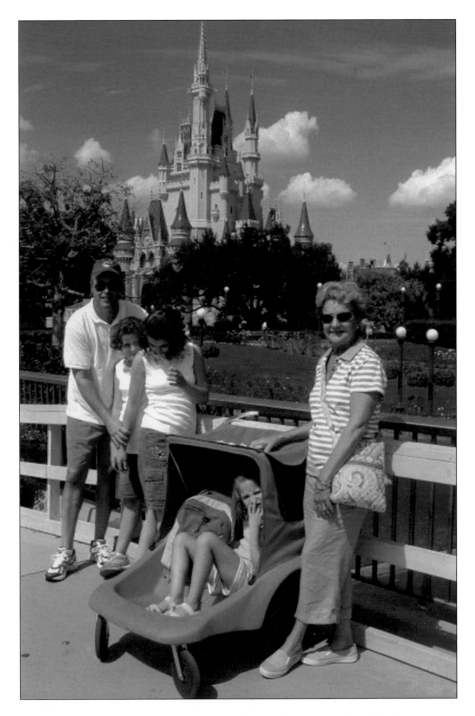

Mark, Gianna, Mia, Bella (in stroller), and my mom, Elena Rossi,
at Disney World, October 2007

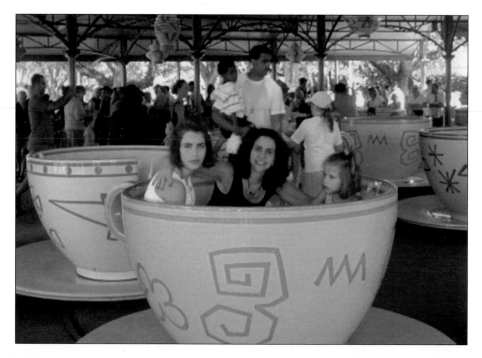

Mia, Kim, and Bella at Disney World, October 2007

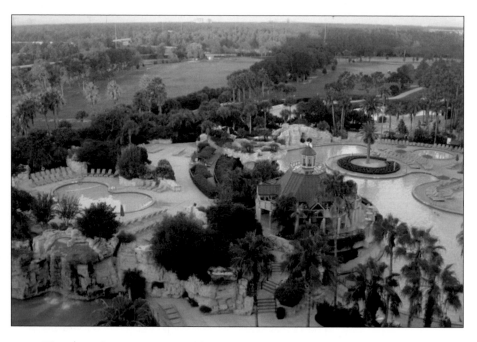

The grounds at Marriott World Center hotel in Orlando where we lost Mia

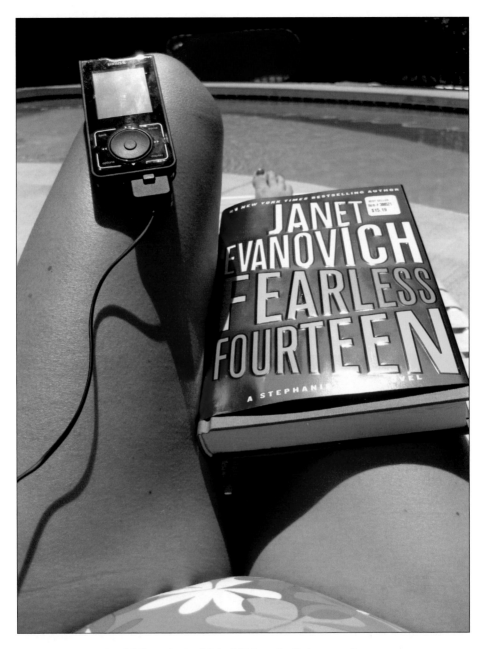

Look! I'm relaxing! July 2008, at the little green house.

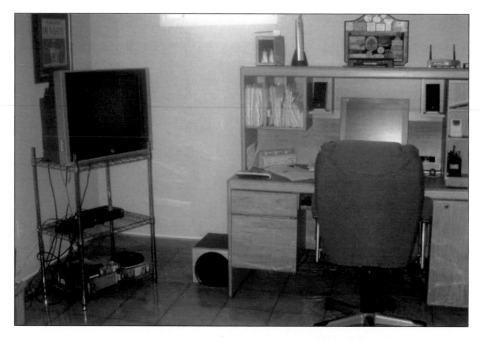

The flood in the little green house. See the water swirling under the chair.

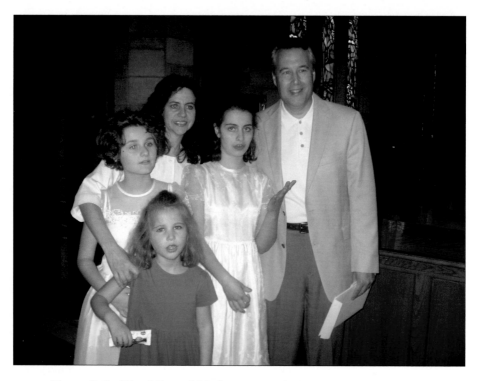

Gianna, Bella, Kim, Mia, and Mark at First Holy Communion, spring 2008

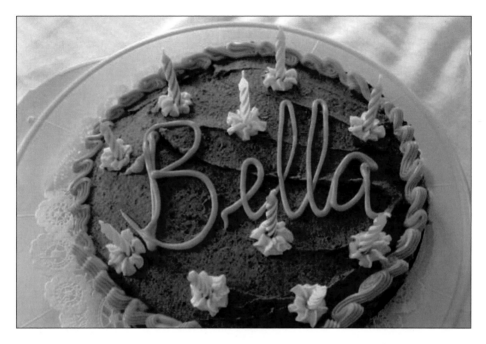

Bella's ninth birthday cake, GFCF
of course, September 14, 2009

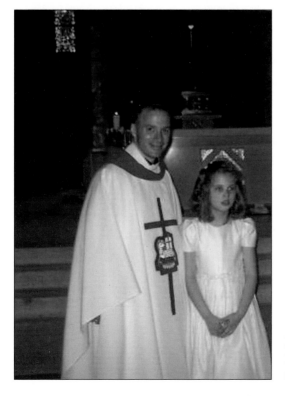

Bella with Reverend Michael L.
Dunn at First Holy Communion,
spring 2010

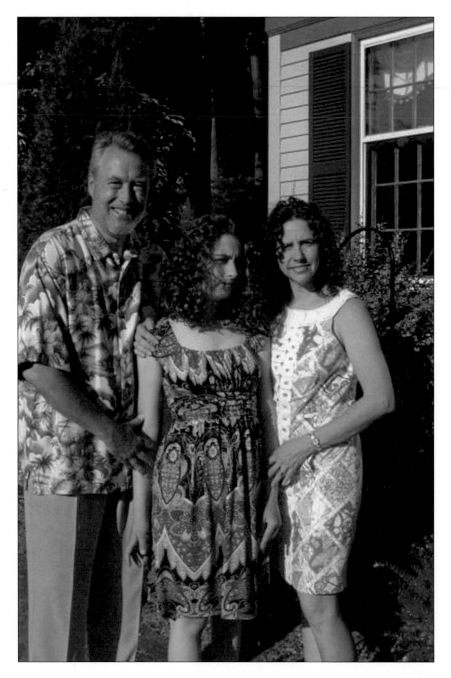

Mia's "Stepping Forth" ceremony from eighth grade to high school, June 2010!

the halls and filled the fridge with store-bought goodies from Heinen's, the gourmet grocery store. We even threw a holiday party, inviting dozens of friends to join us in a celebration. Beer, wine, hard liquor, good food—we had it all!

I was so freaking stupid. And naïve.

By Christmas 2004, I had no more delusions about our future. It looked really grim. We had no money of our own. No jobs. No immediate prospects for work. I still wanted to cobble together a nice holiday for the girls. And I did. Well, it wasn't me—it was the generous parishioners of St. Mary's Church who came through.

Mark and I were placed on a paper mitten on the church Giving Tree by an anonymous holiday elf.

I got a call from a powerhouse of a woman named Kelly in early December. It went like this: "Hi, Kim. This is Kelly. I want you to know that we have your name here at church, and on Saturday you need to come and pick up your holiday gifts."

Me: "What?"

Kelly: "Come to St. Mary's Saturday before 1:00 pm."

Me: "No, Kelly. I mean we're okay." (We weren't.) "Give the stuff to another family."

Kelly: "No way, Kim. You either show up or I'm coming to your house with everything."

By now, I'm starting to cry. Mark and I had dropped off gifts for the Giving Tree every year since we'd been married. We're on the giving team! Not the receiving team!

Holy water, we'd become a name on a paper mitten.

What had happened to us?

I traveled back in time imagining the years of placing a gift for a poor family under the trees at church with the smug (yes, I think I was smug) feeling of a do-gooder.

"Kim, do you hear me? You need this. Do this for your kids." Kelly said.

I mumbled something vaguely affirmative to get Kelly off the phone and hung up wondering if she had just returned from boot camp at Parris Island. As a drill instructor.

Saturday arrived. I had no intention of going to St. Mary's in my $33,000 minivan to pick up charitable gifts to bring home to my 3,200-square-foot, four-bedroom, four-bathroom Georgian Colonial for my family.

Ah, pride goes before the call.

The phone rang. Of course.

"Kim, it's Kelly. *Where are you?*"

Panicking, I looked around my kitchen and at our Christmas tree. My decorations were up, but there were no gifts wrapped and hidden in an upstairs closet.

Kelly's words, "do it for the kids," came back to me.

"I'll be right there, Kelly."

I drove to St. Mary's, praying I wouldn't see anyone I knew. We didn't go to church often, so that wasn't an issue. I walked into the large room where the Giving Tree gifts were stashed.

Holy cow.

There, in a corner, was a pile of gifts, a box of household supplies like laundry soap, a beautiful fresh wreath—so much stuff I could barely fit it in the van. Feeling embarrassed gave way to feeling grateful and excited. Gifts for the girls! I can do just about anything if it's for my kids.

I hugged Kelly and thanked her.

I hadn't told Mark what I was doing, so when I got home and asked him to help me unload the car, he was surprised. We were blown away by the volume of items and the generosity. Together we went through the stuff. There were wrapped gifts for the children, hats, mittens, and scarves, gift cards to local restaurants, an envelope with *cash* in it (must have been from another Italian), movie tickets, household supplies, and the one item that made Mark and me laugh like hell: thirty-six bars of Zest soap.

Did you know that rich people think poor people don't bathe? Neither did I. We may have been down on our luck, but we were Zestfully clean, that's for sure. That soap lasted for over a year, and by the time it was gone, Mark was working. We had a little ceremony as the thirty-sixth empty box hit the trash can. We might even have gotten a little dirty.

NEW WORD: THE STAGTASTROPHE

I was a big fan of Depeche Mode, the 1980s British New Wave group whose songs were not quite as morose as Morrissey's but a far cry from the bubblegum pop of the Material Girl. One of my favorite songs was titled "Blasphemous Rumours." The lyric was, *"I don't want to start any blasphemous rumours but I think that God's got a sick sense of humor, and when I die I expect to find him laughing."*

That sounds about right to me.

We've had so much happen to us since the children were born, I coined a new word, "The Stagtastrophe." We make Murphy look like the luckiest man alive.

I've no idea why I've had so many roadblocks placed in the way of the happy-go-lucky marriage, motherhood, and life I'd imagined for myself as a young woman. Remember those wedding vows?

I'd ordered better, richer, and a side dish of health from the menu of life. We've been served worse, poorer, and sickness at an all-you-can-eat buffet, and frankly, I'm stuffed to the gills and in no mood to tip the waitress.

I take solace in a little delusion I've crafted for myself: "Bad things happen in threes." Well they do, right? Two wizened celebs die a week apart, and the world feigns shock when another 1950s screen star passes away. "See, bad things happen in threes," we tell ourselves, as if to stave off another death. And then—whoops!—there goes another one . . .

The year 2008 was another year of transition for the Staglianos. Finally settled into the rickety yellow house with no front walk and a deck that looked like it was made from timber from the *Mayflower,* we welcomed the New Year with cautious optimism. Mark's job was going well, though there were rumors that financial troubles lurked. His company, NCE Gifts, was the largest wholesaler of decorative flags and had dozens of giftware lines that sold at gift shops, large retailers like Kohl's, and garden centers throughout the United States and Canada. He worked from home, and it was a huge help to me to have an extra set of well-trained (and free) hands available.

Mia was happy in her second year of middle school with Miss Esposito, the difficulty of a new school behind her. Gianna was kicking butt in fifth grade, thanks to Mrs. Windsor and Miss Badowski, two teachers who truly believe that all children are educable if you find the right motivators. Bella was safely ensconced in Miss Saad's first grade, where she was well loved and far more settled in than her kindergarten year. I don't mean to imply that the girls' teachers in Ohio didn't give them 100 percent of their time and affection. They did. But I found that in New England, the curriculum for autism was more specific to the diagnosis. For instance, they used Applied Behavior Analysis (ABA) as a matter of course in school. I should also point out that the teachers in Connecticut were in their twenties, and autism was included in their college training. Plus, they chose to teach the autism population, whereas older teachers simply saw their classrooms transform into autism rooms as the special-ed population grew along with the epidemic of kids diagnosed. It's harder to catch up with the training than to have learned it as a matter of course during your recent schooling.

Even my own career was cruising along—much to my happy surprise. The Age of Autism site was gaining readers every day. We'd made the Google News index, which meant anyone with an alert for the word "autism" got our posts. This was a pretty big deal as it meant our posts appeared in searches alongside an article from

The New York Times or the *Boston Globe*. It expanded our reach, and that's just what we wanted.

I continued to write pieces for the Huffington Post that showcased the travails of autism.

The tranquility lasted for about ten minutes. If you've given birth, think of those moments between contractions. That blessed relief from the pain when you caught your breath and thought that it really wasn't so bad after alllll—here comes another one! That.

I was on the phone with my close friend and confidant Maureen in the midst of our daily (sometimes twice) Verizon to Verizon neighborly chat. She lives in Pittsburgh. Mark came to the bottom of the stairs, looked up, and said, "I just lost my job." My stomach bounced up into my mouth as if I'd jumped over the railing and down to the foyer. Tempting . . .

The Lord giveth to the Staglianos, and the Lord yanketh the rug out from under us. The winter of 2008 was no exception.

Maureen's husband had lost his job in 2006. And she'd helped me through our move when we had to sell our house in Ohio in 2005. She also has a son with autism. She's one of the few people in my circle who "gets" what we've been through from all sides.

I squeaked out, "Oh my God, Mark lost his job. I have to go."

When it comes to sheer terror, practice does not make perfect.

Having been through a twenty-three-month period of unemployment, I was so frightened when I learned Mark had lost this job, I plunged into despair. *That* scared the bejimminies out of me. Kimmy doesn't *do* depressed. Although depression and anxiety are frequent visitors throughout my side of the family. I don't have time for it.

My kids don't care if I'm feeling happy, sad, or am about to take a naked stroll on Route 95 while waving a roll of toilet paper at the traffic. Their needs do not take a break—and neither can I.

I didn't take that stroll on the highway. I drove to church, parked the car, and as I was walking toward the entrance I saw Father Dunn, one of the down-to-earth priests who'd made St. Theresa's such a haven for our family.

"How are you?" he asked.

(Insert flood of tears here.)

He gave me a hug and offered to send up numerous prayers on our behalf. I went inside to ask Mary for help—mother to mother. Then I asked Joseph for help. Father protecting his family. Then I looked up at Jesus on the cross.

"You!"

Yeah. I yelled at Jesus. Then I flounced past the confessional, not remotely remorseful for having called out the Son of God for his shoddy attention to my family's needs and drove home.

I guess you could say I was angry. Fuming. Vesuvian even. How many dues was I going to have to pay in this life?

And I was scared.

If I have one weakness (and I know that I have many) it's that when I'm scared, I become nasty. By nasty I don't mean ten-day-old milk curdled in the carton. Think cornered, rabid dog.

Mark: "I know this is a tough time for us, honey. But it's Valentine's Day next week. What would you like for Valentine's Day, Toonces?"

Angry Kim: "Oh, how about a Whitman's Sampler and a job for you that lasts more than the lifespan of the fruit fly?"

That kind of mean.

Guess what? In six weeks, Mark had a new and wonderful job! You see, when you're good at what you do (and he is, remember that Rookie of the Year award from Lenox China?) people notice. And I assumed that Jesus, Mary, and Joseph and Father Dunn had contributed to our luck.

Mark had been in the wholesale houseware, tabletop, and giftware business since we'd gotten married. He always worked for the vendor, meaning the company that makes (or these days imports) the products. Mark's job was to sell the products directly to retailers like Bed

Bath & Beyond, Williams-Sonoma, and HomeGoods, and also to manage sale representatives from a large national rep group based in Dallas, called One Coast.

The One Coast sales rep in New York had just tendered her resignation to care for her mother, who had Alzheimer's. One Coast had been pleased with Mark's service and professionalism and offered him the rep job with a decent salary. Decent is relative. It was $20,000 less than what he had been making, and still less than what he'd earned way back when in Ohio, but we were grateful. And there was a quarterly sales bonus. Not Wall Street–sized, more like Sesame Street. But we'd take it!

I felt like we'd dodged a torpedo-sized bullet with that job offer. In our Russian-roulette life, the chambers are never empty.

Our landlord was a woman who had moved to China to work for a major U.S. fast food chain. I'll call her "Cathy." She didn't understand why we thought having a stove with four working burners, a dryer that turned itself off, or a dishwasher that didn't try to rinse the floor every time you ran it was a priority. The house had been a pit when we'd moved in, but a few coats of paint and basic repairs had made it livable if not a showplace.

We were sending her what most Americans would consider a sizable mortgage payment every month. On time. Wired right into her banking account. We'd cleaned her filthy walls, painted rooms, replaced dirt and weeds with flower gardens, and added curb appeal to a house that looked like Cinderella long before the makeover.

All she cared about was the money—as was her right. She'd lived for years in the dirty, broken-down house without a care. Different strokes, right?

After the angst of Mark's job situation had faded, I got a call from Cathy. We'd been cordial enough, communicating by e-mail from China to the United States.

She was returning to the United States with a new job that came with a corporate relocation package. She needed to sell her house in order to buy a new house. She told us we'd have to move when our lease expired on June 30. Oh my God, is there anything worse than moving? Okay, maybe moving into a final resting place in the cemetery is worse. But at least I won't have to pack for that one.

One afternoon, I received a rare, chummy phone call from her.

"Hi, Kim, it's Cathy. How are you?"

"Hi, Cathy. I'm fine. What's up?"

"I need to ask you a favor. If a realtor comes to the door, would you please tell her we are relatives?"

Did I mention that Cathy is Chinese?

"Cathy, we don't look like sisters," I said half in jest, fully knowing where she was headed. You see, when you get a corporate relocation package, the company agrees to pay for you to move from your residence. Cathy's residence was in China. Her house in Connecticut stopped being her primary residence and became a rental property the day we signed a lease with her in 2006. I figured the IRS wasn't aware of our lease or the tens of thousands of dollars we'd paid to Cathy. Nor was the company offering the relocation.

No realtor ever came to the door, thank goodness. I'm a terrible liar, and my round blue eyes, curly brown hair, and the distinct lack of photos featuring a single Asian family member would have tipped off a blind man anyway.

I still get steamed when I think of her asking me to lie, and how easily she came by tens of thousands of dollars in relocation payments by her error of omission.

The spring passed quickly. We were into May, still without a new house and a lease that expired in just seven weeks. I was getting nervous.

I called on St. Joseph again, retrieving the statue I'd used to sell our house in Ohio. "Please, St. Joseph, the carpenter who found shelter for Mary when she was about to deliver the baby Jesus, please help us find a house. That's clean. And on a nice street. And in

Trumbull. And under $3,000 a month." I buried St. Joseph upside down in our yard.

And our realtor, Jay, found us a snug, three-bedroom ranch in a basic neighborhood of older homes right off Main Street.

Mark hated the house. I liked it a lot. It had a 1960s retro charm although it was fully updated with a gorgeous kitchen and a master bedroom that felt like a suite at the Ritz compared to the grungy yellow one we were sleeping in. Our belongings would fit right in, which is a real plus when you're renting. You have to shoehorn your life into someone else's house. Our mid-nineties Ivy League–colored furniture (navy, hunter, burgundy) would have looked like hell in a house with a more contemporary color scheme. Most of the rooms were soft yellows and creams, and the kids' bedrooms were pink and white.

The best feature was an in-ground pool with a built-in hot tub in the backyard, with a locking safety fence that cost more than my first car.

Mark walked through the house finding fault everywhere. He hated leaving our 3,200-square-foot house in Ohio (of course, he never had to clean it). It seemed that every house we looked at got a bit smaller and less impressive. But since our next stop was likely to be a tent in someone's yard or my folks' house, I thought the little, green ranch was perfect.

I skittered along behind Mark trying to exude optimism, "But honey, look at this ceiling fan and this pantry!"

I think Mark knew I was at a breaking point. He'd had to stitch his head back onto his shoulders far too many times after I'd bitten it off. The homeowner was renting the house following a divorce. The lack of women's clothing in the closet didn't escape Mark's notice. I'm not sure if that depressed him or gave him hope.

"When could we sign a lease?" he asked.

I winked at the realtor.

Thank you, St. Joseph. And thank you, Mark.

THE THINGS WE DO FOR LOVE

I have a strong sense of Catholic guilt. At my core, I'm honest—someone who tries to make the right choice when presented with a quandary. Sometimes autism and caring for the girls stands in the way of quality decision making. It happens. It's like a man robbing the Piggly Wiggly. When you learn that he's out of work and was stealing diapers for his son, you give him a pass, don't you? (I'm waiting!)

I hope you'll give me a pass.

I've never been arrested, although as the autism world heats up, I think there might be a protest or two in my future that could land me in the clink. Once, I was chastised by the Main Street traffic cop in Hudson, Ohio, for mouthing off to him about a parking situation. Hardly the stuff of *Lockdown*. I don't even park in the "pregnant customers only" spot at the local plaza. I'm waiting for the "customers with an autistic child" spots to appear. I could walk perfectly well, even at nine months pregnant. Navigating my three darlings into a store can be treacherous, though. My friend Connie and I snuck into a firehouse in South Boston and slid down the pole after too many cocktails about a million years ago. Was that illegal?

My brushes with the law were always Lucy and Ethel, not Bonnie and Clyde. Until the summer of 2008, when I broke a Commandment, and not even one of the fun ones.

I was sitting in the yellow house at my computer—just a few weeks before we were to move into the little, green ranch.

★ ★ ★

The kids were upstairs or in their rooms. I think. They weren't under my feet. Mark was out. I was reseaching moving companies online. We were moving across town in a matter of weeks. I was stressed out about the move, worried about how to pay for it, and generally in a bad mood.

A sound caught my attention.

"Plink! Plink! Plink!"

I looked around, glanced at the floor, shrugged my shoulders and went back to work.

Plink! Plink! Plink! Shshshshshshsh!!!!!!

My eyes went up to the kitchen ceiling. Water was gushing out of the ceiling fan (the light was on!) over the movable granite island in the center of the room.

Bella.

OhmyGodOhmyGodOhmyGod, I thought as I raced up the stairs two at time.

Bella had stuffed a Poise pee pad into the toilet. (We used those to prevent embarrassing accidents at school.) The pad had dutifully expanded from a small strip to a bloated, gel-filled pontoon that stopped up the toilet completely. As she flushed several times, the water had poured out of the bowl. How did I know this? It wasn't the first time this had happened. It was just the worst time. The water was now gushing onto the floor, across the bathroom, and had soaked several feet of the hallway carpet. It was at least three inches deep.

Sink or swim, Kim?

I turned off the water at the bottom of the toilet, then splashed to the hall closet to grab every towel and blanket we owned. I could have used a bail bucket. I sopped up as much as I could until we ran out of dry towels, so I began to wring them out in the tub and reuse them. The carpet was destroyed. The baseboards were soaked. Time for damage control. We were moving out, and while I had no love lost for the landlady, I didn't want to trash her house. Always with the guilt.

Mark came home to the catastrophe and just looked at me.

"What the hell are we going to do?"

I'm sure he was imagining a lawsuit or worse. We contemplated for a moment.

"We need a Shop-Vac," he suggested.

"We don't own one, and we can't afford to buy one."

"What the hell are we going to do, Kim?"

Fear not! An autism mom has more badges than an Eagle Scout, and more household hints than Heloise herself.

"I know! I can run up to the Stop & Shop to rent a Rug Doctor carpet cleaning machine. If I use it backward, it will suck up the water."

"You're crazy," Mark responded.

"You got a better idea, pal?" I yelled, as I changed into dry shorts and a fresh T-shirt.

"Lock the bathroom door, I'll be right back. And *don't* kill Isabella!"

I flew up Church Hill Road to the Stop & Shop plaza, slammed the minivan into park, and raced into the store. My cell phone rang and Mark said, "Toonces, get a box fan while you're there to dry the carpet."

Ten-four.

★ ★ ★

I grabbed a cart and whooshed over to the *everything but the kitchen sink* aisle that looks like an Ace Hardware-Staples-Walmart hybrid.

Please let them sell box fans, please God let them sell box—*jackpot!*

I grabbed the biggest fan off the shelf and a small one too, for good measure. I careened over to the self-checkout.

Scan. *Beep!* Scan. *Beep!*

Cash or credit?

I swipe my card.

"Cannot accept card."

Crap. Swipe again.

"Cannot accept card."

★ ★ ★

By now I'm hopping back and forth on one foot like I have to pee the mother of all pees. My ceiling is falling down, my drywall is disintegrating, and my carpet is busy sprouting into a lung-choking strip of death. I do not have time to dawdle. I need to buy the damn fans and go rent a carpet machine. I find a teenage employee.

"What's wrong with this machine? It won't take my credit card."

The kid drawls, "Oh, the card readers aren't working. You'll have to use cash."

Cash? What the f*ck is cash? I haven't seen cash since Ohio, for God's sake.

By now, my armpits are soaked with sweat. I'm doing that thing that my dad does when he's pissed off. It's a sucky sound you make while your tongue rolls around as if you're trying to dislodge caramel from every single tooth in your head. In Rossi parlance it means, "About to blow a gasket, please stand back."

Then the lights dim.

"Attention shoppers. We apologize for the inconvenience, but we have lost power and will have to close the store. Please find the nearest exit."

Now I'm eyeing the Drano in the aisle behind me, and wondering how much I'd have to drink to kill myself right then and there.

No way. I'm not going down. I need the carpet cleaner. I need the box fans. Now.

Move over Lucy, here comes Bonnie.

I rolled my cart, with the two fans inside, over to the Rug Doctor equipment. Drat, it's chained to the display. Off to customer service I go. I recognize the kid working the cash register. He looks like he's in a heavy metal band. His hair is long, his knuckles tattooed, and he has a smile like Antonio Sabato.

"Hi Craig," I say, reading his name tag. "I have an emergency at home, and I really need to rent a Rug Doctor, right now."

"We can't take any money now, there's no power," he says.

God almighty, hasn't this kid ever seen *Little House on the Prairie*? He has a pen and paper, right?

"Craig, I'm in a bind here. Could you maybe write down my credit card information and enter it when I return the machine tomorrow?" I asked in a sweet, slightly strained voice.

"Yeah, I guess I could do that," he said.

Thank God, metal boy has a brain.

He wrote up my order for the machine, I gave him my card info and headed for the door.

The store was in chaos, people still trying to check out, take their groceries, leave their groceries.

I put my head down and sailed out of there as fast as I could.

With my items in the trunk, I eased out of the parking lot and headed home.

Oh no.

I haven't paid for the two box fans.

I pulled into our driveway and schlepped the Rug Doctor from the car to the front door. The house was a New England "garage under," which means it's built into a hill with the garage on basement level. I was not bumping the machine up two flights of stairs. Mark opened the door for me.

"I stole two fans. They're in the car. Go get them."

"You what?"

"It's a long story. Now let's go clean the carpet," I said.

We did manage to repair the house fully. I called an electrician who said the light would be fine—to aim a fan at it for a couple of days and then spray the ceiling with something called KILZ paint.

Sure enough, the light and the fan worked. The ceiling got a fresh blast of paint and the carpet dried out just fine.

No harm. No foul.

Except that I'd stolen the fans. I didn't know if I could go back to the store and tell them. I ended up putting fifty dollars into the Salvation Army's red kettle outside the door as soon as it appeared during the holidays. I told God (because we know how closely attuned he is to my prayers) that I was sorry for stealing them. A few weeks later we had a major flood in our new house, so I'm not sure if God forgave me.

Now you know I've stolen for love. How about public indecency?

★ ★ ★

Our family was in church, and a little boy was seated behind us. I'd visited his family's place for a yard sale last summer (I bought a pumpkin decoration and some manatee books). He was a cute child, well behaved, and maybe four years old. He sneezed. His mom handed him a tissue, and he blew his nose like Louis Armstrong on the trumpet.

Hooooonnnnnnkkkk.

My girls cannot blow their noses. I hate those reminders of how hard it is to teach skills to my girls.

We were once at Mass when Mia had a terrible cold. She hasn't figured out how to blow her nose. I haven't figured out how to teach her. I'm usually pretty good at coming up with some way to relay what she needs to do, but nose blowing had eluded us.

She sneezed, and when I turned to say "bless you, honey," she had the snot equivalent of a bright green eel hanging out of her nostril. I grabbed a tissue and wiped her nose, hoping the other parishioners weren't vomiting in the pews around us. Maybe I'd refrain from shaking hands during the sign of peace? Good plan.

As we left church, I told Mark that I was going to take Mia to the urgent care center, as it was obvious that her cold had turned into a sinus infection.

The waiting room was busy on a late Sunday morning. Mia and I sat down and waited for her turn. She was quite patient. Up to a point.

"Bathroom?" she said to me.

When any of my kids indicates the need for the toilet, I drop everything and take her. I put down the clipboard and took Mia to the restroom. She didn't go.

★ ★ ★

Back in the waiting area, she said it again, "Bathroom?" Up we jumped, only this time, I noticed a small wet stain on the back of her jeans. My heart sunk. I didn't want her to be embarrassed. When my girls get sick, they can't always feel when they have to go in time. This was one of those times. We went into the bathroom.

"Wet!" she said to me.

Mia, like any of us, doesn't like the feeling of wet clothing. You and I don't strip off our clothes, however. If she became agitated she might want to undress in the waiting room. I looked at her. She was so beautiful, with her dark hair and big eyes. I felt so sad.

"Wet!" she said again, kicking off her shoes and starting to undress. Oh boy, I had to think fast. Mia needed dry underwear.

Lightbulb!

"Hang on, Mia. Mama will fix it." I told her.

In a jiffy, I'd slipped off my own shoes, wriggled out of my jeans, and pulled off my underwear. It felt like being in the mile-high club, except the toilet water wasn't blue, and I wasn't having any fun.

★ ★ ★

"Here, put these on," I said, as I held my underwear down by her feet. She stepped into them and got dressed. I grabbed my jeans, thanking God I hadn't worn my favorite white Levi's, and carefully slid them on, zipped them up, and ran a mirror check.

Together, we went back into the waiting room. Mia was snug and dry. Me? I was going commando.

A good friend will give you the shirt off her back. A good mom will give her child her underwear.

THE LITTLE GREEN HOUSE

We moved into the darling ranch house across town on July 1, 2008.

Gianna was turning twelve on July 11. She'd made friends for the first time in her life in the Trumbull schools. I invited ten little girls from her regular-ed fifth-grade classroom to a pool party.

I also broke down and bought Costco cupcakes loaded with gluten and topped with colored sprinkles. Gianna's eyes nearly popped out of her head.

"Wow. Giant cakes for Gianna! I love it!" she said.

The party was the first in our new house. I loved the kitchen, which had a green granite countertop, stainless-steel applicances made in Germany, and a "beverage" fridge with plenty of room for wine and beer.

And the pool? Wow. Once they were in the water, my girls' differences just melted away. Mia and Gianna can swim thanks to "drown-proofing" goals on their school plan, which ensures they get swimming lessons once per week. Bella can't swim yet, but she can float like a demon in a safety ring.

You'd never know my girls were autistic while they splish-splashed away an afternoon. I have a great photo of Mia and Gianna with several typical kids, holding hands, about to jump in the water.

I even took a self-portrait lying by the pool with the newest Janet Evanovich "Stephanie Plum" book on my lap (covering my middle-aged, three-kid stomach) just to have proof that I'd actually relaxed during daylight hours. (Sometimes I look at that photo like it's a relic from an archaeological dig.)

It's nearly impossible to take the three girls to a public pool. Mia is our indoor cat, and she's anxious to go home within half an hour of our arrival. Bella loves the water and will sit and splash at the water's edge for hours. Gianna will either swim or pace around the pool, asking if her friends from school are coming. Inevitably someone has a meltdown. Bathing suits get yanked off, in public. Screaming is not out of the question.

When Coppertone makes SPF Invisible, we'll be much better off.

Having a private pool was beyond decadent.

★ ★ ★

Then a harbinger of new problems appeared at our front door.

Have you ever seen a "dunning letter"? Neither had I. Despite our financial ups and downs, Mark and I have always paid our bills on time. For poor people, we have really good credit scores. (We can thank his mom for helping us out financially during that long bout of unemployment.)

Tucked between the screen and front door of our little green house was a letter from a bank, requesting that the homeowner contact them immediately. I knew enough to realize this did not mean there was a shiny new toaster waiting for our landlord, whom I'll call "Angelo."

A few days letter, I opened a piece of junk mail without checking the name on the envelope:

Bankruptcy doesn't have to mean you can't have a new car!

Oh. My. God.

Our new landlord was late on his mortgage and bankrupt to boot?

This stuff could only happen to us.

We knew the house was part of a divorce situation. But in our naïveté, it hadn't occurred to us to run a credit check on the landlord.

I Googled "bankruptcy Connecticut" and found an automated phone system that provides basic details on bankruptcy filings. Bankruptcies, like foreclosures, are public record. I called the number, punched in Angelo's name, and sure enough, the son of a bitch had filed for bankruptcy on *Gianna's birthday!*

Then *another* bank left a notice in our mailbox. Two mortgages!

I asked him about the bankruptcy.

"Don't worry," he told me. "It's just my ex-wife's credit card debt." Sure. Did she shop at The Men's Wearhouse and buy thousands of dollars' worth of landscaping equipment for *his* failed business? (Those were just two of the creditors on his bankruptcy filing. You can check all that stuff at the courthouse.)

Did he think I'd just fallen off the zucchini truck? I'd been hearing horror stories on the news about marshals showing up on doorsteps and evicting unsuspecting tenants throughout the country! Can you imagine if that happened to us with three autistic kids?

When I saw that first dunning letter, I worried. And then I set aside Angelo's money woes and went for a swim. *Que será será.*

Fall came, and the little green house demonstrated another fine feature. We could sit in the front room and watch the bus approach through our front window, then let the girls skedaddle down our own brick walkway to the waiting bus. (The yellow house didn't have a front walk—just grass.)

Mia and Gianna started boarding the bus by themselves. A new skill.

As the holidays approached, I started to feel at home for the first time in more years than I could remember. I hadn't realized just how homesick I'd been for New England until I'd returned.

President Obama had won the election, and optimism was in the air. In a nod to my newfound (and much appreciated) sense of security, I unpacked my Lenox china for the first time in almost five years. It brought back so many memories, mostly good. The hope and optimism of our wedding day. Serving our first married Christmas dinner. The Christmas I didn't eat a morsel because Mia was having seizures all day. I said mostly . . .

Do you recall that torpedo that missed us when Mark found a new job? Well, it struck us broadside in a direct hit.

It was early November, and I was planning my Thanksgiving dinner. I, like every other American woman who is not an acolyte of Paula Deen (fry it) or Martha Stewart (hatch it, raise it, slaughter it yourself in the backyard), "plan" a basic roasted turkey with traditional fixings.

I was seated at my desk, when I heard Mark snap his fingers behind me.

I turned.

He had his phone to his ear, his face was chalk white, and he simply made a cutting motion across his throat.

Holy freaking moly, he'd just been fired. Again.

I think the right word for the sound that came out of my mouth is "keening."

I dropped to my knees and sobbed.

He hung up the phone, and said the worst words I'd ever heard from him.

"I'm so sorry, Kim. I've let you down. I'm so sorry."

And he wept.

My heart broke. I knew what a good job he'd done for the company, but retail sales had dried up as gas prices skyrocketed and the economy went into a death spiral. His accounts had simply stopped writing purchase orders.

We were financially at the end of our rope. We'd saved some money, but then used it earlier in the year for the couple of weeks he was unemployed and to pay for our move (which cost more than $2,000—moving our kids quickly and with as little disruption as possible necessitated the cost.)

We clung to each other for a moment.

"Don't you dare apologize to me," I begged him.

Within hours Mark had his résumé out to several headhunters and was making those agonizing phone calls he'd made only months earlier: "I'm out of work. If you hear of anything . . ."

I sent an e-mail to my family and closest friends. *Mark lost his job. Economy tanked. Half of sales force let go. Don't call me yet. I can't talk to anyone.*

Dozens of colleagues rallied around Mark. A testament to his reputation.

We got through Thanksgiving and marched toward Christmas. This marked our third holiday season in five years with Mark out of work. You'll laugh, but I was sort of grateful that the girls' autism prevented them from asking for age-appropriate gifts. It would have broken my heart to tell them, "No, we can't afford a Wii" almost as much as it hurt to keep supporting the Sesame Workshop by wrapping yet another Elmo toy every year.

I both started and finished my Christmas shopping in the Stop & Shop: broccoli, Tide, plastic Elmo cell phone. I kid you not. I spent less than a hundred dollars on the three girls. I told my extended family I'd send them millions of holiday wishes but not much else.

December 2008 was a cold month.

And wet.

I usually start my weekdays at 5:30 am I make coffee, log on to my computer to check overnight comments on Age of Autism, prepare three gluten-free breakfasts and lunches, and get the girls ready for school.

On the morning of December 12, Mark helped me and then headed to his office in the basement. Down the stairs he went.

One, two, three, four, five, six, *splash*!

"Oh my God, Kim! We have a flood!" he hollered up the stairs.

I ran to the door and peered down the six steps into the basement. Clear water was running across Mark's feet on the basement floor. A monster storm had hit the night before, and, while we were sleeping, the sump pump had decided it was time to die.

Mark climbed back up the stairs. We stood on the top step looking at the swishy swirly water. He shook his head.

"We're effed."

"How are you not dead?" I asked him finally, aghast. "The lights are still on, and everything is underwater . . ." my voice trailed off. I'm no fainting Freida, but I felt woozy at the thought of how close Mark had come to electrocution.

My husband had stepped into several inches of water in a room where submerged power strips were loaded with the electrical cords of a humming office. If any reader is an electrical engineer (or a priest?) and can tell me why Mark wasn't electrocuted when he stepped into the water, drop me a line. I call it a miracle.

I thought I'd gotten past caring about "stuff." I hadn't. Despite being grateful that I was planning a cleanup, and not Mark's funeral—my framed portraits of the girls, our wedding pictures, my in-laws on their wedding day, my grandparents, everything, everything, everything we'd kept in boxes down there was ruined! Not to mention hundreds of dollars' worth of empty boxes we use for moving. Clothing. Books from my childhood. All destroyed.

Even Mark's golf clubs (tee hee!).

My brother Rich and his partner Ed had splurged and sent the girls an expensive *Sesame Street* kitchen for Christmas. That kitchen had become a galley—on the *Titanic*. I saw the water swirling around the white box from Amazon and lost it. My kids had one good Christmas gift, and now it was gone.

But, like most Stagtastrophes, this one passed, and we managed to count the very big blessing that Mark had not been injured. Angelo immediately replaced the sump pump, and the water drained away, leaving behind muck and our soaking-wet belongings.

One of those "like it never even happened except your stuff is gone" companies came and dried out the entire basement, carting away hundreds of pounds of sopping-wet boxes. Our insurance agent had included sump-pump coverage on our renter's policy. (Thank you, Doug!) It covered $5,000 of the estimated $8,500 we lost.

Christmas approached and with it a renewed hope in the goodness of people. The autism community reached out to us from all directions. A dear friend and mom of three kids on the spectrum (one of whom lost his diagnosis due to her hard work), the fabulous Michelle Iallonardi, took up a collection and sent us a check for more than $1,000 and a scarf her mom had knit. The National Autism Association called to offer us a Helping Hand grant of $1,500 to help pay for the girls' supplements. A Yahoo group for old-timers in the autism world sent me a box of all sorts of goodies. An anonymous donor from New York City sent us a thousand-dollar American Express gift card! It bought our groceries for months.

I was overwhelmed with gratitude. How did so many people love us?

We were even a paper mitten on the giving tree for the second time.

One night close to Christmas, our doorbell rang, and when I looked outside, Santa's elves had left a large gift bag loaded with goodies for our family.

There was a box in the package labeled "for Mom." In it was a gold bracelet with diamonds and sapphires (to match my engagement ring). I wear it every day to remind me that we are never alone.

It's humbling to accept help with grace.

I've learned to say thank you, swallow my pride, and remember that every gift is sent with love and concern.

★ ★ ★

The year 2009 arrived. I'd turned a year older just before New Year's Eve. We settled in for a long winter's ... work. We don't get many naps here. January brought the excitement of the inauguration of President Barack Obama, whom both Mark and I had supported. It also brought continued reports of the worst economy since the Great Depression.

Mark had been on a couple of job interviews. But for all intents and purposes, the job market in his industry (and every other) was stone-cold dead. We had enough money to last until April. Just a few months away.

I was back to feeling scared. And that meant I was back to feeling angry.

At one time I'd had a plaque with that saying from Mother Teresa: "I know God will only give me what I can handle. I just wish God didn't trust me so much." (I'm pretty sure I sold it at a garage sale.)

I was starting to wish that God would just forget about me for a while and concentrate on something else, like a plague of locusts, or maybe a famine.

Mark had continued to receive calls from vendors and colleagues in his industry. First one, then two, then three vendors asked if he'd continue to represent their product lines. Before he knew it, he had a company. It was strange. It was improbable. He'd always been with a corporation, and I'd liked it that way. We needed the benefits for the family. But as everyone knows, benefits are nonexistent today. No 401(k) and we still had to pay $998 a month for our "company-sponsored" health insurance.

Mark discovered he *had* a job. He was self-employed.

I liked to say that the only person who could fire him now was *me*. Not that I'd ever get rid of the rock that anchors our family.

April came and went. We limped along financially. My generous sister and brother stepped up to the plate and helped us meet some of our expenses. My eighty-six-year-old father pulled me aside at Easter and told me we always had a home with him and my mom— who had a habit of tucking "a little something" into a card of encouragement on a regular basis.

I was getting excited to open the pool and enjoy another summer by it.

Angelo the bankrupt landlord had other plans.

One day in spring he called and told us that an appraiser was coming to the house. Oh boy. Again I asked, "Are we okay here? Is the house okay?"

I saved his voice mail: "My attorney is on top of it. You have nothing to worry about." Right-o, Angelo!

The appraiser came. I introduced myself as Kim Stagliano. I could see the mental lightbulb go on.

"Are you a tenant?"

"Yes," I answered. "And I know that the landlord is bankrupt. If he's appraising the house, does this mean he's about to lose it?"

The appraiser was circumspect and shared no information. If only I'd been in my bikini when he'd answered the door. Of course, then he might have run away.

I knew that having him at the house didn't bode well for our being able to remain as tenants. And I loved that little green house.

Lo and behold, in early May, Angelo alerted Mark that he would not be renewing our lease at the end of June.

I called him. I was furious.

"Angelo! We talked about staying on here for at *least* two years when we signed the lease!"

"I know, Kim, but I need to move back in so my girls can go to school in Trumbull. My ex-wife is leaving town."

Off went my bullshit meter. *Whatever* the reason, Angelo needed to move back into the house. Oh God, how were we going to manage another move, two in one year! My mind began the checklist of dread: Get new boxes, pack, try to prepare the kids and keep their anxiety levels below code red, call moving companies, cable, electric, gas, fill out more change-of-address cards, and on went the list. I was exhausted on top of being really angry at Angelo, whom I felt had really snowed us.

I went into action. What else could I do?

"Hi, Jay?" (our realtor at Coldwell Banker.) "It's Kim."

God bless Jay. Realtors make no money on rentals. But Jay called us every day with listings and showed us several houses at the drop of a hat. He's a doll.

★ ★ ★

Mark and I walked into a lovely Dutch Colonial and smiled at each other. It was a mile from the middle school, walking distance to Starbucks, and the rent was equal to what we were paying Angelo. Within a week we'd signed a two-year lease *and* learned that the house was paid for—no landlord worries!

Because of the December flood we had far less stuff to move. How's that for a very pale silver lining?

We try to take each tumble off the horse as it comes. We've climbed back into the saddle more times than I can count. Sometimes I land on my backside, but I've never landed on my head. I'm always okay. My kids are happy. My husband is by my side.

And that is what I call "Stagtastic."

THE MIDDLE CHILD

My personality has helped my ability to cope with this crazy life. I didn't go from a shy girl who never raised her hand in class to a thinner version of Roseanne just because of autism.

In kindergarten I can remember making fun of a girl named Shirley for wearing baby shoes—they were white sandals with a covered heel. They were a safe, appropriate shoe for a five-year-old. I told her she looked stupid in them.

In first grade, to avoid drinking my ice-filled half pint of milk (can you stand ice in your milk?), I'd lie to Mrs. C., "I'm going to upchuck. May I be excused?" Then I'd dawdle in the hallway until an eighth grader would spy me, haul me into the bathroom, and make me do my notorious Fat Albert imitation, "Hey, Hey, Hey!"

Sister Barbara nicknamed me "Hot Seat" in third grade because I could-not-would-not-did-not sit still. I'd race through my work and then bounce up to find something more interesting than my desk. If I were a kid today, a doctor would have me on meds for ADHD. I'm still pretty willy-nilly. That's a major frustration for my über-organized husband.

My nickname in fourth grade was "Bossy Rossi." In seventh grade I wrote an advice column called "Ask Kim." We printed it on the mimeograph machine (I'll give you a second to remember the smell of the chemicals that clung to the damp copies that thing churned out, if you're old enough).

For some reason, I was voted class president in eighth grade, as a newcomer to the school. I'm still not sure if that was a joke or if I'd made an impression on the class in two short months. Maybe they elected me to spite another student.

Even as a kid, I had "leadership" qualities. But the autism world has some deep rifts. And not everyone thinks I'm the cat's pajamas.

For instance, there's a group of self-advocating young adults and adults with autism (many of whom are self-diagnosed) who dislike the autism treatment community because we want to change our kids' autism. Hello? My girls can't cross the street safely. These folks can blog their hatred of me and talk about me all night on chat groups and blogs. I'd hardly say they share my kids' problems, although I've no illusion that any form of autism or Asperger's is a walk in the park. With the unusual abilities and talents often trumpeted come depression, isolation, employment problems, and sometimes an inability to live independently. And, boy, some of them are pissed off about the seach for an autism "cure."

The irony is that their own autism prevents them from empathizing with what my girls deal with every day. I can deal with these folks because I always imagine how happy I'd feel if my girls were *able* to start nasty blogs and devote all their time to dissing some mom in Connecticut and her peers.

Then there are the skeptics who attach themselves to autism like barnacles. Skeptics are the folks devoted to debunking what they see as myths, including the autism-vaccine connection. I've no idea why this is so important to them. To me, it's like attacking the folks at Mothers Against Drunk Driving for wanting to prevent drunk-driving-related deaths. Stupid.

But boy they are a busy little group of bees. They hide behind online pseudonyms or use the fourty-fourth–fifty-second digits from Pi as their screen name and then they comment over and over and over and over and over and over (feel the perseveration?) on posts about autism and vaccines. There's one dingbat on Huffington Post with 30,000 comments who claims to be a mom in the Midwest. Honey, if you've had time to comment 30,000 times on a blog, someone had better call child services, because your kids must be really hungry. I suspect they are financed by pharma. Others just want to deny what may have happened to their own children. The anger is way over the top and the nonstop assault they put up is absurd. They never comment on my softer "mom" Huffington Post pieces. I guess they don't get paid for that.

★ ★ ★

The most nefarious are the autism "experts" who are hell-bent on making certain that autism is not viewed as an epidemic, and who advocate the position that it is not treatable, let alone curable. At the risk of sounding like that tinfoil-hat model, I have to wonder if the lack of medical attention to autism outside of genetics and a handful of frightening psychiatric drugs stems from the realization that *all treatment roads* would lead to an eventual determination of cause. The cause *could* include vaccines.

The December CDC announcement that was so underreported stated that the autism prevalence for eight-year-olds has increased again to one in 110 children. That's almost one percent of children! The numbers have jumped from one in 500, to one in 250, to one in 166, to one in 150 and now to one in 110 in just a decade. And that 110 estimate uses data a couple of years old. We could be at one in *under 100 kids.*

At what point should we panic about autism? In my house, the panic train left the station a long time ago.

One of the so-called experts in autism is Dr. Fred Volkmar from the Yale Child Study Center, which is about fifteen miles away from my home. He had the audacity to claim that media awareness is behind the increase in autism. Check out this bit of an interview in Medscape:

Medscape: Do you think the increase in autism is mainly due to the expanded definition?

Dr. Volkmar: It's a couple of things. First of all, there's more public awareness. The fact that we're having a discussion like this, twenty years ago nobody would have ever called me to talk about autism. It's partly the media and it's organizations like Autism Speaks and other things for good or bad. Even on the Internet, if you type in autism into Google, you will get 15,000,000 hits. The trouble is, only about 100 of those are worth anything and of that 100, about one third are quite problematic. There's more information, there's more media attention, there's more public awareness. We now get referrals from day care providers, who in the past wouldn't even know what the word meant. It's much more in the public conscientiousness.

Is he completely bananas? The reason no one talked about autism is that they weren't affected by it. I'll bet that my eighty-eight-year-old Uncle Mortimer didn't jabber on about prostate issues when he was thirty. Does Dr. Volkmar really think parents whose kids can't speak or provide the most basic self-care only got noticed recently because Autism Speaks ran some public service ads telling parents that their kids had a better chance of having autism than playing for the New York Yankees?

Fred Volkmar blames the increase on the media and the autism organizations that have cropped up in a desperate effort to help families. Got it. Right. Okay. He's the expert, after all—Yale, you know. Big doings there! Lots of funding. Well spent, don't you agree?

When you have an autism leader saying an increase is in doubt, even as school resources are being overwhelmed trying to manage and educate the autism population, I get very, very angry. Then I start writing. And then get I those icky Google alerts.

A thick skin doesn't grow nearly as fast as you'd think. I'm still working on mine.

Perhaps more than others, I need to be liked by people.

Ah yes, the middle-child syndrome. I blame it for my incessant desire for attention. I credit it for my sense of humor and ability to make people laugh. I was a classic class clown.

★ ★ ★

A bit about my sister and brother:

My older sister Michele was beautiful (still is) and the object of everyone's attention. She looks like an exotic Snow White. With my oversized eyes and round cheeks, I looked more like Dopey. She's four years older—which feels a lot better in my forties than it did when I was four. We had a good relationship as kids. She left for boarding school when I was in seventh grade. I followed her to the same school the year after she graduated.

When I was a freshman (called IV class in prep parlance, and yes, the Roman numeral makes a difference, much like adding the suffix "pe" to "shoppe" inflates the bric-a-brac prices), I was sitting at a carrel in the library, and there scratched into the desk were the words MICHELE ROSSI IS BEAUTIFUL. It was my very own Jan Brady "Marcia, Marcia, Marcia" moment. I used my left hand to scribble "All Rossi's are great," assuming no one would know that it was my own (ridiculous) comment. Was I a loser or what?

I can barely describe how unattractive I was when I began high school at the age of thirteen. My brown hair turned from wavy to American Standard Poodle overnight. I wore a thin cloth headband with the little grosgrain ribbon on top. In 1977, it made me feel like I fit in with the preppy crowd. Today you'd be ridiculed for placing it on your Chihuahua.

I wore giant glasses with blue plastic frames and blue-tinted lenses that hid my best feature, my blue eyes. And they had a gold letter K sticker on one lens. Hey, Laverne looked great with an L on her sweater, why couldn't I have a golden initial sticker on my eyeglasses? Because a thirteen-year-old's eyeglasses are not the same as a busty adult woman's chest, perhaps? That part was lost on me. Speaking of busty, I was thin and flat chested. Aw heck, I might as well share this little fact: I used to wear turtleneck dickies—the quasi-shirt that goes over your head and covers your chest and back with two flaps. I figured out that I could increase my bustline by tucking the front material up and under my Sears bra. I've no idea what the boys might have thought come spring when I shed layers and a cup size. I'm pretty sure no one noticed at all.

Upon graduation, I followed my sister to Tufts University. By age seventeen, I appreciated her popularity more than I envied it. Plus, having blossomed to a full A cup and having learned to straighten my hair, I was less competitive with her. I even joined her sorority house.

Twenty-eight years later, I remain a Chi Omega pledge. I never formalized my membership in the sisterhood, having hightailed it out of Tufts for Boston College my sophomore year, allegedly to study business.

In reality, I wanted to be on the Green Line of the MBTA transit system, which offered me a straight shot to Arlington Street station around the corner from where I caught the Vermont Transit bus to visit my boyfriend Dave at Dartmouth. At Tufts I had to ride a bus into Harvard Square in Cambridge, take the Red Line to Park Street, and then transfer on the Green Line to Arlington Street. Not exactly a well-thought-out reason for changing colleges, I admit. Have teen decisions ever been well thought out? I only thank God and Jesus I didn't have a camera phone back then. Enough said. My mom and my priest are going to read this.

I loved Boston College, though, and graduated in 1985 along with a famous autism dad named Doug Flutie.

Back to the middle-child angst.

My brother Richard is the youngest and the only son. He was born on Valentine's Day, 1970.

I spent the next twelve years tormenting him for having the audacity to join our family. Buried in a family photo album is a snapshot of little Richie dressed in the white pantaloons and floral pinafore worn by my three-foot-tall Raggedy Ann doll. Michele and I painted his face with green eye shadow and turned him into a Martian once, too. He was adorable with his sandy-blond hair and chubby cheeks. I can still picture him sitting on the Pawleys Island hammock near our house taking his first sip of the drink that I, his loving big sister, had offered him on a hot summer day. The cup was filled with pickle juice.

Despite my initial jealousy of his existence, I grew to love him, even though I'd gone off to boarding school when he was seven years old and didn't see him daily. Lucky for him, right?

When Richard graduated from The Catholic University of America in Washington, D.C., he came out to my mom during a walk to the lake down the street from our childhood home. Soon after, he called me on the phone to tell me he was gay. I was standing in the spare bedroom of Mark's and my apartment on Cross Creek Trail in Brecksville, Ohio. I can't imagine how hard that call must have been for him. I wasn't shocked. It was good to know for certain, though, after having the idea nibble around the edges of my consciousness for a few years for the usual reasons. He'd had no dates or amorous mentions of girls. And he went dancing to techno music at the clubs on Lansdowne Street in Boston while wearing rubber shoes.

★ ★ ★

I finally knew for sure that Rich's roommate Ed Wood was more than just a roommate. Nineteen years later, Rich and Ed are still together, and in my mind are every bit as married as Mark and I, or Shelly and her husband, Mike, or my parents, despite the discrimination they face regarding marriage.

My dad, who was born in nineteen hundred and twenty-two (that's how he says it), accepted my brother and Ed. I will always respect and admire my dad for that. My mom's main concern was always for Richard's well-being. She worried about AIDS. She worried about discrimination. She grieved the loss of having a daughter-in-law and grandchildren "the traditional way." She never expressed worry to me about how having a gay son would reflect on her and my father.

My mom and dad taught me how to be a parent. They've been married for over fifty years. My parents' example of love and acceptance is why I've been able to cope with our challenges and remain married to Mark. I've no idea what keeps him with me except the bitter realization that being in your fifties, financially starting over, and having three kids with autism isn't the trophy wife magnet a man might think.

Whether it's the blessing of my middle-child syndrome or not, most people seem to appreciate my ability to add humor to a pretty grim topic. They seem to appreciate that I'm an outspoken mom, willing to put myself (and my family for better or worse) in the public eye. Even those who don't agree with my autism causation and treatment opinions will tell you I'm a "good mom." I try to reach out to others and build bridges where I can, despite disagreements. Sometimes I'm good at it. Sometimes I fail. Sometimes I'm in a snit and I don't bother to try at all—preferring to lob a grenade on Huffington Post or Age of Autism. The results of these grenades can be found all over the Internet: "Kim Stagliano's writing is pathetic" pops up on an obscure blog, and my stomach clenches. I've been called a bitch, a disgrace to journalism (I'm not a journalist and have never claimed to be), a rotten mother, and more. Nice, huh?

I won't stop chronicling life with three gorgeous girls with autism, even if I never get used to the criticism.

Luckily, I have my family to support me.

I wonder if my brother is up for a visit anytime soon? I'd better check to see if I have any pickles.

UP, UP, AND AWAY

On October 5, 2009, The American Academy of Pediatrics journal *Pediatrics* confirmed that the autism rate is now one in 110 children. Flags are not at half staff. The military is not in the streets. The mainstream media is showing signs of Xanax overdose in their reporting. No worry. Not a hint of panic. No hard questions as to why so many kids are neurologically impaired.

However, just a month before the *Pediatrics* study was published, a study came out from the National Health Service Information Centre in the United Kingdom that claimed the rate of autism among adults, according to their calculations is—drumroll please—one in 100 *adults*. That dovetails with the new American numbers better than the drawers in a Stickley dresser, doesn't it?

If you can convince the public that there are one in 100 *adults* on the spectrum, perhaps that's *always* been the rate of occurrence, even in America. Then you don't have an epidemic of a severe neurological disorder—you have better counting.

It appears that our doctors, mainly pediatricians, have simply gotten much better at recognizing and diagnosing youngsters who cannot speak correctly or at all. Who have socialization problems. Who would sooner look at the pattern in the floor tiles than their own mother. Brilliant, these doctors, aren't they?

Let me tell you—my childhood pediatrician, Dr. Germain, would not have missed autism in me or my siblings. *Dr. Doolittle* couldn't have missed autism.

★ ★ ★

Ah, Dr. Germain. I can still see his crew-cut hair and quick smile. I can feel his chilly hands. He terrified me, of course. I don't think doctors felt compelled to be terribly friendly in the 1960s, Marcus Welby notwithstanding. Dr. Germain demanded, and commanded respect. He had a paddle over the entrance to the examination rooms. On it was a painting of a boy and a girl bent over at the waist, with the words, "Board of Education." What's more shocking is that there wasn't even a Pfizer logo on it! Ah, good times seeing the pediatrician in 1969. He was forthright, direct, and smart. He would not have missed autism, even if he doubted what he was seeing due to its rarity at the time. And he wouldn't have been afraid to break the bad news, an excuse I hear often today about our pediatricians.

While I'm not quite in AARP territory, I'm no youngster. In fact, there was a song written to celebrate my birth, "Late December 1963 (Oh, What a Night)." All right, it was about some other special lady, but I was born on December 28, 1963, and the song made me smile as a kid—even though that special "night" would have been about nine months earlier for my parents.

I'm trying to remember which of my peers in my school, neighborhood, town had autism, or even Asperger's. I'm quite familiar with how those diagnoses look. I'm pretty sure I'm as good as a pediatrician at recognizing the signs. You can go grab a cup of coffee while I calculate the vast numbers of kids from my childhood who were affected.

Back so soon? I'd barely reached my eighth-grade classmates at Mercy Mount Country Day School in Cumberland, Rhode Island.

★ ★ ★

I remember Lonny Kane, who was a young adult with cognitive disabilities in my town. Lonny would have been labeled "multiple handicapped" in a school system today. I would guess that he had cerebral palsy and cognitive challenges. The kids at school made fun of him. Including me and my tap and jazz dancing pals from The Young Sophisticates School of Dance (we were as sophisticated as kids could be eating Funny Bones, drinking Fresca, and dancing to the theme from *Rocky* in a town called Plainville, Massachusetts.)

I happen to be a stellar voice impersonator. I had Lonny's tone and cadence down to a science. I even squinted my eyes, bucked out my teeth, and contorted my posture. Ha! I had the full Lonny!

God, I was a mean kid. Worse, I was a mean kid with leadership qualities. And I didn't give a rat's patootey about authority. A charming combination. And yet, it's worked to my advantage as an adult struggling to help three children with autism. Go figure.

How rotten was I as a kid? How's this for being no Mother Teresa?

★ ★ ★

I always had to be the first to complete a test, to win the race around our small Catholic elementary school building, to do things better than my friends. I was better at getting in trouble, that's for sure.

In sixth grade (I was all of ten years old, having started first grade at five) my "boyfriend" Jack and I went on a field trip to the John Hynes auditorium in Boston for the Whole World Celebration. Whole World? We stuck with Russia and Cuba—he had packed a flask of vodka and cherry cigars. Of course, a Sister noticed my booze breath on the bus home and called my parents immediately. I was suspended from Dominican Academy for a few days.

Can you imagine what my parents thought of me? They must have been terrified I was on the fast track to Skid Row. Well, Mark and I did end up homeless, so maybe that wasn't a stretch.

As you can see, I'm not prone to shame—in fact I'm rather immune to it by now, having had enough autism moments with the girls to hold my head high under the most alarming circumstances.

I am ashamed that I made fun of Lonny. He didn't choose his lot in life. And I didn't do anything wonderful to end up neurotypical.

His parents were loving and kind and at his side every time I saw him. My mom told me Lonny's mom died, and his dad still takes care of him. Mr. K. must be quite elderly by now. It foreshadows my girls' future.

I have a second cousin about my age named Dawn who has profound cerebral palsy. She is a twin. I saw her sister Debbie several years ago at a family reunion. It pains me now, as an adult, that I didn't know her better or make an effort to understand what she was going through. I wonder if this is how my own children's cousins will feel about my kids? It's difficult to get to know my girls—due to geographic separation and the family quibbles and general life issues that distract us all. I worry that I should be training these boys and girls, my nieces and nephews, to love and look out for their cousins who did not dodge the autism bullet as deftly as they did.

Up the street from us lived Steve Welsh, who had Down syndrome. Always quick to grin, Steve now lives in a gorgeous Nantucket-style group home his mom had built on her own property. My mom still sees him in the area and he's doing well. His mom doesn't realize it, but she's a beacon of hope for me—I worry greatly about what will happen to Mia, Gianna, and Bella as Mark and I age. Seeing that Mrs. W. built a home for her son (and others) quite literally in her side yard gives me hope that we'll find creative, safe, and loving living options for our girls.

So that's three people with disabilities in the first twenty-one years of my life; none of them had autism. None of my friends had a sister or brother who was "institutionalized" as often happened back then.

When I graduated from Boston College in 1985, I went to work as an Assistant Account Executive at Hill, Holliday, Connors, and Cosmopoulos Advertising in Boston. I rode the bus from Newton Corner to the John Hancock Tower in the Back Bay. There was a man on that bus whom I believe had autism. He was about 5′7″ and had dark hair with bangs that fell down his forehead. He was a bit chubby and walked with a rolling gait. He could see, but his head moved around like Stevie Wonder's and his eyes usually looked upward. He had a man with him, perhaps an aide or another sort of paid helper. I remember thinking that the helper was a terrific guy for hanging with this poor soul. At the time I was a twenty-one-year-old YIT (yuppie in training) wearing Belle France dresses to work and dining on turkey and Boursin herb cheese sandwiches at Au Bon Pain each day. I looked at this man as a tragic figure—but not much more.

A few years ago, when I learned that there were people questioning the idea of an autism epidemic, who believed we simply had better diagnosis, the image of this man on the bus whose name I never knew burst into my memory. The only words I ever heard him utter were, "It's Wednesday! It's Wednesday! It's Wednesday!"

★ ★ ★

Calendars can be a source of fascination, perseveration, and perhaps routine comfort for people on the spectrum. My daughter Gianna is very in tune with the calendar. I can ask her on any given day, "Gi, what day is it?" and she'll tell me.

By the age of twenty-one I had come into contact with a person somewhat older than myself who had autism. One person. Not one of my friends in grammar school, junior high, or prep school had a sibling with autism.

One of my dear friends is Ginny G., who, as a teenager, was my babysitter. I'd told her boyfriend at the time that he was ugly. What an angel I was. Ginny attended teachers' college and went into special education. I've had long talks with Ginny about her career and what she knew about autism back in the early seventies. In a nutshell, she was taught that autism was rare. And she saw only a handful of students with the diagnosis.

Ginny is now a grandmother of three little girls and a grandson. One her granddaughters has an autism diagnosis, Pervasive Developmental Disorder—Not Otherwise Specified (PDD-NOS). Another has some sensory issues.

Ask any special education teacher over the age of forty-five how many kids with autism they had in their classrooms, whether in public school or the old state school systems back before inclusion was an option, and they're going to tell you, "One. Two. None." Now go ask a special education teacher who's been teaching for five years the same question and then stand back.

I recently struck up a conversation with two women while seated at the bar waiting for a table at a restaurant on Cape Cod. Mia had sort of gotten in their faces with her greeting, which can startle people. She rubs her hands and puts her face close to yours and makes a humming noise. The two women were very kind to her. When we were seated, I thanked them for being nice to Mia and explained she has autism. Their response, "Oh, we knew, we're former teachers." I seized the opportunity to ask them if they'd seen many students with autism during their careers. "One," said the first. "No," offered her friend.

When Autism Speaks came onto the scene in 2005, the rate used by CDC was one in 166, recently up from one in 250. That was a huge jump from the numbers in the 1970s and 1980s. Then in 2007 the number increased to one in 150. Now, in 2009, the number is a confirmed one in 110.

Today, we have entire schools devoted to teaching children on the spectrum. Tomorrow we're going to need high-rise apartments to provide safe residences for many of them. I'm hopeful that a good number will recover and lose their diagnosis, going on to lead full, independent lives, get jobs, and pay taxes. It seems the young kids who are being diagnosed today are responding well to intense therapy and treatment. That's a bit of hope in an otherwise depressing circumstance.

We become immune to numbers. Five soldiers killed in Iraq. (I'd like a Venti latte). Another child was beaten to death by a peer in Chicago. (Did you watch *Mad Men* last night?) One in 110 American children has autism.

Do you care?

DON'T ASK. DON'T TELL.

A Couple of years ago, I was on a panel at Elms College in Chicopee, Massachusetts. John Elder Robison, who wrote *Look Me in the Eye* about his life with undiagnosed Asperger's growing up in the same household as his brother Augusten Burroughs (who wrote *Running with Scissors*), was the headliner. I was in the chorus, and just happy to share the stage with him. He's one of my favorite people, and my first adult friend with Asperger's.

How I survived forty-three years without running into a whole lot of Aspergians is beyond me, considering the drumbeat in the media and some research circles to convince the world that autism, in its myriad presentations from low functioning to Aspergian savant has always been with us at the current rate. Autism can include a person who doesn't speak and appears to be severely mentally challenged, living in his or her own world, rocking back and forth, and someone like John Elder Robison, who has had several successful careers, is articulate, is probably a genius, and who lives what most of us would call an enviably comfortable, "normal" life.

Heck, I worked for one of the geekiest high-technology companies in America and cannot recall anyone on the spectrum there. That company was Bolt Beranek and Newman, in Cambridge, Massachusetts. With apologies to Al Gore, BBN is the company that really did help create the Internet; they designed the "Arpanet" for the United States Army in the sixties.

I'd just been fired from my position as an Assistant Account Executive at Hill Holliday Connors & Cosmopulos, purportedly due to budget cuts on one of my accounts. I think it was because I screwed up a media insertion and ran a full-page major product announcement ad for Lotus Development (remember Lotus 1-2-3 software?) in the *Wall Street Journal* on the *wrong day*. Ouch.

I wish they'd been straight up with me about why I was fired; I could have learned something other than humiliation and how to apply for unemployment. I now know that firings rarely come with explanations. I sure didn't ask them for details. I just trudged home, shell-shocked.

Anyway, my friend's mom needed a new assistant at BNN. Her old one had just left to work at Boston Technology making some pie-in-the-sky new product called "voice mail," which no one was ever going to use, what with the ubiquity of the pretty young receptionist in every corporate lobby in America. I had high-tech marketing experience and so she hired me. After working at Boston's largest ad agency, joining BBN Software was akin to being in charge of watching paint dry for Sherwin-Williams.

BBN Software made a product called RS1, a number cruncher for manufacturers. Their glitzy product was ClinTrial, which ran statistical analyses on pharmaceutical company clinical trials. The place should have been crawling with autistics, eyes averted, mumbling about trains, and lining up the peas on the cafeteria trays.

I can remember the product manager who used to sit/stand/ mount the edge of his desk, posing in a manner he might have thought was provocative. The young female marketing team thought he was repulsive. I can see the face of the VP of marketing, who later lost his job and appeared on a national program about the difficulty of finding a new job when you're over fifty. I got to know his pain all too well twenty years later. And I'll never forget the wonderful, larger-than-life gal whose water broke in the bathroom—turning me into an instant midwife as I escorted her down to a waiting ambulance. ("God, please don't let her get that stuff on my new shoes!")

I can't recall a single employee with autism. And my memory is very good. That doesn't mean they weren't there, so don't go sending me hate mail. Perhaps they were not in visible positions.

Today, when I go out, I often find that other family with an autistic child. It's like having gaydar for autism. Do I ask them about their child? Do I tell them about my own?

I hesitate to do more than make eye contact with the parent, smile, and nod. You never know if the child has a diagnosis or not, and I'm sure not going to spill the beans to a mom or dad who hasn't heard the fateful words yet. For starters, I'm not qualified. Am I accurate? You bet. Most of us in the autism world can spot another child from across the mall.

You just know by the walk, the face, and the way the parents act around the child. Sometimes the smile and knowing nod leads to a conversation. Kind of like a foot shove under the stalls in the men's bathroom. Except not quite so intimate.

While the autism epidemic took off in the 1990s, there *are* older people with autism. I don't want to imply that I believe otherwise. That's disrespectful to the parents who've come before me and fought like heck so that my girls can attend school and have services.

Last summer, Mark and I had taken the girls to Sunny Dae's ice cream in our town. We brought our dairy-free ice cream for Bella and digestive enzymes for Mia and Gianna, ready to enjoy as typical an outing as is possible. Taking the kids into any public location is like herding cats, but we manage, and the familiarity of Sunny Dae's is easier than trying someplace new.

I sat down with Mia and Bella, while Mark and Gianna went to place our order. At the next table was a beautiful woman, with patrician cheekbones, a sweep of dark hair, and an elegant countenance. Next to her was an equally beautiful younger woman who instantly reminded me of Mia. How can I describe what tipped me off? Well, she was at one with her ice cream. I don't mean that she was messy or inappropriate, she simply was concentrating on her treat to the exclusion of her mom seating next to her. She just had "the look." A bell went off in my head; *Whoop! Whoop!* Autism at twelve o'clock!

★ ★ ★

The woman and I made eye contact and smiled at each other. The dance began. She spotted autism in my girls as fast I recognized autism in her own. At that point, it's a matter of who leaves the gate first. I did. Of course.

"Hi, this is Mia and Bella. Mia reminds me of your daughter. Does she have . . ." I try not to label my kids or others in public where they can hear me. The mom knew what I meant.

"Yes, she does," she answered, with a European accent.

"My name is Kim Stagliano, it's nice to meet you."

"My name is Sophia Moldavi."

"I know you, Sophia, we've e-mailed each other many times!"

Sophia runs an organization in Greenwich, Connecticut, and is creating a farm for adults with autism, like her own beautiful daughter. She gives me hope and scares the hell out of me at the same time. Her daughter is approaching forty. I can barely think to when Mia turns twenty.

That brings me to a question I've been asked: "If you suspect a child has undiagnosed autism, do you tell the mom or dad?" I've already given you my short answer. "No." But that's not completely accurate. I did once tell a parent.

★ ★ ★

I was at a Silpada Jewelry party at my neighbor's house in Hudson. The night before, Mike G., the handsomest dad in the neighborhood (next to Mark, of course), was walking while pulling his young son in a Little Tikes wagon. I was in the driveway when he walked past our house. I heard him say, "Use your words, Jay!" in a stern, exasperated voice.

My heart dropped.

I knew the family and that the boy was having difficulty with behavior. His dad just told me that the boy also had autism.

I flashed back to a park in Doylestown when Mia was maybe seventeen months old. She loved to swing, like most toddlers. I'd give her a push while saying, "Push, Mia!" with a big smile on my face—willing Mia to talk to me, not just at me. I'd let the swing stop, hoping Mia would tell me to push her again. She could speak. She had words. I knew that she could say "push."

But she wouldn't utter a sound. She just stared at me. Her eyes that so closely matched my own, were blank, as if telepathy was enough for her.

That was one of my first warning signs that all was not well for Mia. And I'd used the exact words with her that I'd heard Mike say to his son: "Use your words, Mia!"

★ ★ ★

Mike's wife, Cheryl, was at the Silpada party. She was a special education teacher and a damn good one. But like the doctor who smokes, sometimes when a situation hits so close to home, it's hard to see. Cheryl is a beautiful woman, with sleek, blond, coiffed hair and perfectly applied makeup. At that party, her face looked pinched and her eyes tired.

Should I tell her? What would happen to our friendship if I shared my concerns? What would happen to the child if I did not?

I quietly approached her and said, "I heard Mike walk by with Jay last night. He sounded really frustrated. I wanted to ask you if you've considered maybe having him tested for an autism diagnosis?"

Then I waited. Would I get a glass of white wine thrown at me? Would she slap my face? Storm off in a huff?

"You know, Kim. I have. And I'm so glad you mentioned it. . . ."

Wow. From there we had a really good talk. Cheryl is a great mom to Jay. And Jay is doing well. He has Asperger's Syndrome, is a funny kid, earnest to a fault, smart as a whip—and getting the services he needs.

★ ★ ★

Today, in my position as a writer and blogger, I get e-mails from strangers, "My grandson isn't talking, and he's almost two. The pediatrician says it's because he's a boy, but I'm concerned." I want to bang my head on my desk when I read that tired response from doctors.

On one hand, experts tell us better diagnosis is behind the rising autism rates. On the other hand, I'm still hearing from parents and loved ones of kids who are clearly not developing properly that they struggle to get a diagnosis.

I try to answer as gently as I can, without instilling false hope. "Trust your gut," is my usual answer. "Don't jump to conclusions, call Early Intervention, check out the GFCF diet for GI issues," rounds out my suggestion.

Sometimes the call or e-mail is not from a stranger. Those especially make my heart sink. Like the twenty-seven-year-old woman whose wedding Mark and I had celebrated just a few years ago, who e-mailed me a laundry list of issues in her seven-month-old that made my knuckles turn white on the computer mouse and my heart drop. The child had severe reflux, could not eat, had not learned to sit up or roll over, and was not babbling.

"What do you think, Kim?"

First off, I admired the mom for having the balls to ask me. That's a good sign, for the child most of all. Mom isn't hiding and is taking her daughter's health into her own hands.

But honestly, how do you answer when someone you care about says, "What do you think?" Am I supposed to be honest and say: I think the child is on the bullet train to Autismland? I could never say that to a young parent. Hope is too important. Not denial—hope. There's a difference.

★ ★ ★

Autism is a frog-in-the-pot diagnosis. The water heats up around you and then starts to burn. It's not my place to plunge mom into that pot. With enough intervention, a child can fight off or lose the diagnosis. I'd rather get Mom started on progress than simply scare her to death.

We don't know what medical advances there might be in just a year or two. I want Mom to get cracking and feel productive, not despondent.

I suggest Web sites like the National Autism Association and Talk About Curing Autism (that alone gives Mom some idea of what I'm thinking) and I try to point her to some experts in her area including Early Intervention. My goal is to help, not to horrify. I know that by the time a young parent has asked me for my opinion, she's already aware of a problem. But every developmentally delayed child does not have autism. Although, when I hear about severe GI problems along with gross motor and speech delays, I see a red flag the size of a football field.

In addition to better diagnosis, we're told autism is genetic. In fact, I'm often held up as the "poster child" for the genetics of autism, because all three girls are considered on the spectrum. Let's take a look at the Rossi Stagliano genetics. Mark's siblings have four boys and two girls between them. My sister has one son. There's no autism, even in the boys. There have been some scares—a seizure disorder in one, a strange fainting syncope in another, some weight issues for a couple—but I'm grateful none of the Stagliano sibs or my sister has to go through what their brother and I and their nieces live with every day. All of these kids are smart as whips and excellent students. I know my girls are smart, too—I just don't know why they fell to autism.

I realize that ten kids do not make a proper statistical sample (see, my time at BBN Software paid off) but even when I expand up the branches of our family trees, there's no autism in sight. My dad is one of nine children. I have over twenty Rossi cousins. No autism.

My mom's mother, my Grandma Yoli (short for Yolanda), was one of ten children. My grandmother was alive when Mia and Gianna were diagnosed, and while she was not well educated, she was sharp and bright and never had a single story of an "odd" relative who may have been sent away to a home like the Kennedy child named Rosemary. My mom is one of four children who collectively have six children of their own. No autism. Even among the second cousins, there is no autism to be found. On Mark's side of the family there are also dozens of cousins, both Staglianos and Mackeys. No autism.

Genetics only? Better diagnosis only? No way. That's nothing more than a patronizing pat on the head.

★ ★ ★

I'm going to ask *Why, What, How,* and *Who* until my voice is raspy and my fingertips bloodied from pounding the keyboard. What caused my girls to become autistic? Why is no one else in our family affected?

"Don't ask, don't tell" doesn't work for the U.S. military. And it sure doesn't work for autism.

ANOTHER NIGHT IN THE HOLIDAY INN EXPRESS

I wish this were a chapter about taking vacation. If it were, then I'd make another wish—that it was about staying at a fancy Ritz-Carlton or Four Seasons hotel, no offense intended to the Holiday Inn Express chain. And as long as I was wrapping myself in champagne wishes and caviar (yuck, make that choco-late) dreams, just Mark and I would be at this luxury hotel, looking out the window of our suite at the Eiffel Tower, lit from top to bottom on a clear Paris night. Of course, if any of that were true, I'd be reading someone else's book, not writing my own.

With an autism diagnosis, every day is another day in the Holiday Inn Express, where you have to become the expert whether you have a GED or a PhD.

In 1999, when Mia and Gianna were diagnosed in Cleveland, Ohio, we didn't get a treatment plan of any sort. We were told to continue with the public schools, because the girls were three and four years of age. We did that, and the girls got some benefit from being among other children and receiving an hour or two of speech and occupa-tional therapy a week. I had never heard of Applied Behavior Analysis (ABA) therapy for autism. And the folks at University Hospitals of Cleveland were handing out autism articles a decade old, so they weren't exactly a go-to resource for current treatment. Our wealthy suburban school district, like many, was just waking up to the need for autism programming in their system, and they didn't offer ABA.

Because of this, for many years I didn't think ABA was very valuable. In fact, I shunned it. Had my girls been diagnosed in California, ABA would have been built into their school program without my having to ask. And they would have made more progress and learned more skills before entering kindergarten. I'm not big on regrets, but I can admit to mistakes. I should have pursued ABA for them.

I didn't do much better with Bella. Early Intervention in Summit County, Ohio, was sketchy, and my growing mistrust of medical and school services stood in the way of taking advantage of the programs they offered. The kind woman who did our intake mentioned that Bella might have mild cerebral palsy. That nearly stopped my heart. I could handle developmental delay. I knew autism. CP? No.

I was an idiot.

I should have let Early Intervention give any and every service to Bella, if only to engage her and keep her little body limber. Mia was in the throes of her seizure disorder, and I left Bella to her own devices (motherly euphemism for I ignored her) far too often.

There's a wonderful writer/journalist named Karl Taro Greenfeld. His older brother Noah has classic autism, and his father, Josh Greenfeld, wrote three books about Noah in the 1970s and 1980s. In 2009, Kart wrote a follow-up book called *Boy Alone* about what it was like to grow up with a sibling who was profoundly disabled by a disease that was virtually unknown at the time.

I had the pleasure of meeting with Karl for a few hours one morning in New York as he was writing his book. I read his dad's three books before our meeting.

★ ★ ★

I was blown away by the fact that so little had changed within the autism world since Noah had been diagnosed. Close to forty years had passed, and I, upon getting my girls' diagnosis, was in the same position that Karl's parents had faced decades earlier.

No treatment plan.

No hope.

No cure.

Karl's parents took matters into their own hands, finding every treatment they could for Noah. If you've read *Boy Alone* (and you should), you know that Noah remains within his profound autism despite the intense treatment and the love of his parents, who I consider the very first Parent Warriors. Karl faced the decision that thousands of Americans will confront in the next decades as caretaker for an adult sibling with autism along with aging parents.

He moved his family from New York to California to care for his brother, in an act of unselfishness few will be able to match.

Into the new millennium, I and countless other parents had to do the same thing as Josh and Foumi Greenfeld—blaze a path for our kids using whatever tools we could find or afford.

The young parents I meet online and at conferences have more access to information thanks to the computer. Jenny McCarthy calls it "attending the University of Google." But that doesn't necessarily make life any easier, as it's nearly impossible to sift through the treatment choices, analyze them, figure out which ones might work best for your child and how you can pay for them—all while taking care of a child who is likely a difficult toddler.

There are books galore on every sort of therapy and treatment. Most of the options are expensive. Few are covered by insurance. Even as states add insurance mandates, I'm not hopeful they'll stick. Once Aetna and United Healthcare and Kaiser realize they have to spend $50,000-plus per year for a child with autism, I fear they'll find a way to unload our kids from their plans. Diagnoses will likely slow down as doctors are told to put the brakes on the financial strain of autism on the insurance system. Kids will suffer.

★ ★ ★

To muddy matters further, the treatment communities themselves are at odds with each other. The ABA-only folks cling to the "scientifically proven" label like a life preserver, despite studies that show ABA is not a panacea. The biomedical treatment folks (my crowd) has its own share of zealots, some touting treatments that make even a veteran like me roll my eyes as I imagine dollars swirling down a drain.

A diagnosing doctor will probably tell you that your two-year-old needs twenty-plus hours of ABA a week, because of that "scientifically proven" label. Good luck obtaining that level of service in any strapped Early Intervention program, or finding and funding it yourself. A couple of years ago, when Mark was actively looking for a job, I spent a lot of time on Monster.com trying to help him. I ran across a job in Massachusetts that depressed the heck out of me. A family was advertising for a full-time ABA therapist for their youngster with autism, and the salary was $50,000 a year. Can you imagine paying $50,000 a year out of pocket?!

★ ★ ★

Let's say a parent chooses to see a doctor who specializes in the medical treatment of autism—a doctor from Defeat Autism Now!, part of the Autism Research Institute in California that was founded by Dr. Bernard Rimland, who also was a cofounder of the Autism Society of America. (Generation Rescue also has a list of doctors who are treating autism.) You'll walk into the office full of hope, as these doctors are treating the medical conditions that accompany autism, and some of their patients are dropping the diagnosis. You'll walk out of the office a couple of thousand dollars lighter when you account for the visit, lab work, and prescriptions and supplements you'll need. Can you afford to spend that kind of money? Your child's future is at stake. Can you afford *not* to?

Back in the days of home equity loans, easy credit, and padded 401(k) accounts, these decisions were a bit easier because you could find the money to pay for the options you selected. When the econ-omy tanked and so many Americans lost jobs, those cash sources turned off like wells gone dry. This has only added to parents' frustration.

I'm sure parents whose kids have other serious diagnoses, like cancer, muscular dystrophy, or cystic fibrosis, also have to make a whole lot of agonizing decisions on behalf of their child. Some of those may involve life and death. As much as I worry about my kids, I know that they are basically healthy and well. I can kiss them goodnight, every night, and know that the next day, they will awaken. I don't take that for granted.

★ ★ ★

On the flip side, I think there's less tolerance, understanding, and sym-pathy for my kids and for the autism community in general. We don't have a Ronald McDonald House or Make-A-Wish Foundation. When was the last time your church or synagogue organized a fund-raiser for a child who was just diagnosed with autism?

When I gave birth to Bella, Mark and I ate like a king and his queen for two straight weeks with hot dishes appearing magically at the door nightly at five o'clock. Five months later, when Mia's sei-zures began and I was struggling with two youngsters with autism and a newborn, the phone never rang, the doorbell was silent. Playgroup moms do not sign up to make a month of homemade din-ners so that mother of a newly diagnosed child can have a break.

As a parent, I want the public to know how tough autism is for the entire family, most of all for the kids. I want Autism Speaks to stop running ads showing towheaded boys in Abercrombie outfits looking sad because they will never play baseball for the New York Yankees while standing alone on a cul-de-sac in New Canaan, Connecticut. I want to see a twelve-year-old boy in the middle of a rage. I want the world to see the mom who has a fat lip from her daughter who lashed out during a sensory meltdown. I know far too many people who clean feces off their walls every single day and whose children sleep on a plain mattress on the floor, not in a bedroom that looks like a page from the Pottery Barn Kids catalog.

This is the reality of autism for thousands of families.

* * *

To their credit, Autism Speaks has shown the underbelly of autism, in the movie *Autism Every Day*. And they took heat from many high-functioning folks with autism who were offended by the portrayal of parents struggling with their kids.

On the flip side, I don't want people to hear "autism" and either fear or hate our kids. There has been a spate of newspaper reports of crimes and arrests where the word autism is thrown into the head-line like chum into the water. Autism is not synonymous with vio-lence. Autism does not mean "danger to society." Soon after Seung Hui Cho, the angry student who strafed the Virginia Tech campus with bullets, killing thirty-two people, the rumblings began, "Did he have Asperger's?" I immediately wrote a Huffington Post piece decrying the quick assumption among so many.

I've made a cancer analogy in the past and have taken heat for it. I don't give a crap. Autism is like cancer. Not literally, but in terms of *perception*. Let's say your father calls you on the phone and says, "I found out today that I have early stage prostate cancer." Now imagine if he said, "I found out today that I have pancreatic cancer." Those two sentences invoke a different set of assumptions. Prostate cancer is treatable. You hang up the phone and worry. Pancreatic cancer is a death sentence. You hang up the phone and vomit.

How do we walk that tightrope of wanting the public to under-stand the good, the bad, and yes, the ugliness of autism, while maintaining respect and dignity for our loved ones? They need help, not hatred. God, I'm starting to sound like a bumper sticker.

* * *

Autism has become a blanket term for every inch of the spectrum from the most severely affected to the highest functioning success story with Asperger's. I think that's a mistake. It denies the gravity of diagnosis for many, and could paint someone like my friend John Robison with the wrong brush.

Welcome to the Holiday Inn Express known as an autism diagnosis. Don't forget to tip your maid. Checkout time is at . . .

DOES HEROIN FEEL
THIS GOOD?

Today is January 4, 2010, the first day of school after the interminable holiday break. Yes, interminable. As in, "Mommy loves you, but, my God, are you children still here and where *is* that school bus?" I cannot fill ten days of break with meaningful, engaging playtime or work time for three children with autism. I cry uncle!

Because God really does have a sick sense of humor, we had a 90-minute delay for cold weather today. Cold weather? We live in Connecticut, not North Carolina. Twenty-degree weather and blue skies on the Monday we finally, finally, finally get the kids back to school does not say, "Oh stay home for another hour and a half, kids!" to me. However, I don't make those decisions. Perhaps the superintendent got a Snuggie for Christmas and simply couldn't bear to un-Snug himself at five thirty this morning.

Telling my girls that we have a school opening delay means nothing to them. When they wake up, they wake up. There's no settling back down into the bed for another hour. For any of us.

I don't blame them for being eager to go back to school. School is much more fun than home. Mia kept saying, "Time for Miss Jianine. Time for Miss Laura." Gianna was gearing up for her after-school Connections Club and for swimming class on Tuesday where she could play the new game she made up. "The drowning game." Yeah, Gianna is using her imagination, which is a huge leap forward for a child on the spectrum. She invented a game where she drowns and her friend Vicky has to save her. She spent weeks last Fall saying, "Vicky! Vicky! Help! Gianna is stuck!" before I finally asked her teacher what on earth had happened in the pool. Hey, she was alive. She had not drowned. I wasn't that concerned. With autism you have to choose your worries with care. The report back from school was, "It's a game she made up. She pretends to get stuck and Vicky frees her." That's fabulous progress. But really, couldn't the next game be something a little less Addams Family and a bit more Cleaver? Nah, not in our household.

Bella, meanwhile, my sweet little Bella, spent much of the vacation heaving her purple Land's End backpack at me, which was every bit as effective as saying, "Ma! Get me back in school!" Hint taken. I'd put the backpack into the front hall closet. She'd retrieve it and hurl it at me. Ah, good times, holiday break.

By 9:27 this morning (but who's keeping track?) all three girls were safely on their buses on their way to school.

A-freaking-men.

"This must be what heroin feels like," I thought to myself as I closed the front door and made a beeline for the coffeepot to see if there was any left. It was a new year, and things were good.

On December 15, 2009, Mark got a commission check that would choke a horse. A small horse. Okay, more of a pony than a horse really. For us, anything bigger than an unemployment check looked damn good. It meant we'd survived the worst financial year we'd ever faced. And the pipeline, now opened, was going to flow freely with steady income.

We had the best Christmas I can recall in years. And not just because we had a few shekels to buy presents. My sister's stepsons, Mac and Sean, decided to spend Christmas with Grandma and Grandpa in New England and flew in from Texas. This meant that for the first time, we were all together in my childhood home. Mark, the girls and me, Shelly and Mike and their son Colin, plus Mac and Sean, Rich and Ed, and my parents. My dad is in his late eighties. It was such a blessing to be together at the end of what had been a really tough year. My folks couldn't stop smiling.

Christmas morning arrived. Mark handed me a jewelry box. I hadn't seen one of those since our ninth wedding anniversary in 2000. (I can't count the paper mitten bracelet given to me by the church angels in 2008.)

Inside was a pair of diamond earrings in a design called The Everlon Knot. *"The Everlon Knot is the strength of love forged in an endless unfailing knot. It is a symbol that even in the toughest of times— especially in the toughest of times—the strength of your love will never waver."*

Perfect.

The Everlon Knot is a marketing ploy, of course, created to convince men it's okay to buy jewelry even in a bad economy. I'd considered myself impervious to ad campaigns for jewelry, like those silly right-hand diamond ring ads, *"For me."* But those Knot ads got me. What woman wouldn't fall for this after the years Mark and I had weathered?

I placed the earrings into my ears and admired the sparkle in the mirror, thinking that Mother Teresa was right. God will only give you what you can handle.

But it's really nice when your husband gives you diamonds.

I'm wearing the earrings now as I'm listening to Howard Stern and wondering where Artie Lange has gone. Most of us fans assumed rehab, since there was no death announcement, and he's an admitted heroin addict. I guess that's why I have heroin on my mind this morning. I don't do heroin, in case you're wondering or my mother is reading this. Never have. The only white powders in my house are Johnson and Johnson Lavender, Bob's Red Mill Arrowroot, and Clabber Girl cornstarch. Promise.

I wonder what I'll do with my kid-free morning. Maybe read a book. I read several memoirs over the last year or two. I wanted to channel some of the magic into my own book. (Of course, I've written a Kimoir, not a memoir. Isn't that catchy? It makes me feel less old. You can roll your eyes if you'd like.)

I avoided depressing memoirs and stuck with memoirs by comedians, to see how they balanced the funny and the heartfelt. I never wanted this book to be maudlin, or as my dad would say, a "Me poor lady" book. I want understanding, mostly for my kids. I want help, entirely for my kids. I do not want pity. My life may be different from what I'd expected, and my kids' issues are severe, I get that. But I'm happy. Genuinely happy. I wouldn't trade my girls for three little Olympians or *American Idol* wannabees, or the smarty pants kids who get those letters saying that because of their stellar performance on the state tests, they've been invited by the Abe Lincoln Foundation to travel to Australia to study the habitat of the Aboriginal Boola Boola bird if I'll please just send in a $3,000 deposit. Don't laugh. Mia has gotten that letter every year since fifth grade because the schools modify the state test for her. One of these years, I'm packing her bag and sending her to the airport just to see what the tour guides will do. I smell a civil rights lawsuit!

Sarah Palin's *Going Rogue* was not on my list of "must read" books, despite its popularity. I prefer to laugh *with*, not *at*. I read Kathy Griffin's *My Life on the D List,* Howie Mandel's *Here's the Deal: Don't Touch Me.* Neither made me want to pop Prozac like Certs, which struck me as a very good thing. Both made me laugh out loud.

I could hang with Kathy Griffin. And she'd like me, because even though she is older than I am (meow) she looks a lot youn—well, maybe not younger, but a lot more plasticky than I do, and that implies youth, which is good enough for many women.

Later that January I was in Trader Joe's shopping for groceries. A little boy who resembled that itty-bitty chicken hawk kid in the Looney Tunes cartoons (big head, short, glasses) looked up at me as I pawed around for gluten-free waffles and said, "Hi. I'm four years old, and my name is Noah."

(Kids who do not have autism boggle my mind.)

I looked straight at him and said, "Hi, I'm forty-six years old, and my name is Kim. Happy New Year, Noah."

Not sure if his parents were tickled pink at their son's precocious introduction or horrified that I answered him. They hightailed it over to the organic yak milk.

DR. WAKEFIELD AND
THE ANTI-VAXXERS

(Good name for a chapter about the autism/vaccine controversy. Bad name for a Motown band circa 1968.)

Lately, my "Kim Stagliano" Google searches turn up the phrases, "anti-vaccine" and "anti-vaxxer." Despite the fact that I vaccinated my two older girls fully when they were younger and have never told a parent, "Do not ever vaccinate your child," I have been branded with the "anti-vaccine" label.

It's a great label if you want to make a quick point and box me into a mythical category for a sound bite. "Oh, Kim Stagliano? She's that anti-vaxxer lady who runs that 'anti-vaccine' Web site called Age of Autism." It's the equivalent of calling those who are pro-choice "pro-abortion baby killers," even though many folks who are pro-choice, like me, are personally pro-life. As long as we're going down Controversy Street, let's take a left turn into Abortion Alley for a second.

Mark and I had one of our favorite priests over for dinner on a Friday night. As I stood at the stove, I felt like Carmela Soprano, who used to cook for her priest to compete with the other ladies from church. I prepared eggplant and veal parmagiana and baked a chocolate pistachio cake, Mark's favorite.

I had never invited a priest into my home. He arrived at our front door wearing a pair of jeans and a sweater. No collar. He's a regular guy with a quick wit. That he can perform the Last Rites in case you keel over in front of him is a plus, too. He blessed our house and gave the girls three beautiful pink crosses that now hang on our walls.

Because I am incapable of normal conversation, I managed to weave abortion into our dinner conversation. Thank God Mark knows the Heimlich maneuver. (Kidding, Father Dunn is used to my blunt talk and even managed to swallow a bite of veal and a very large swig of wine as I was talking.)

Here's my abortion story: The doctor who delivered Isabella also delivered Mia six years earlier, when we first lived in Cleveland, Ohio, prior to moving to Bucks County, Pennsylvania. We had an excellent relationship, which is to say that I had a monstrous crush on him. He was handsome, charming, South African (oh, the accent), and partially responsible for ending the agony of labor and making sure all my parts were back in their right place after delivering Mia. What's not to love?

Dr. P. had a son with severe ADHD. I had two very young girls newly diagnosed with autism, which I told him about at my first prenatal visit. He had firsthand knowledge of the difficulty of raising a child with neuro issues. In fact, he knew far more than I did about what I was facing. At that visit, he said, "You know, Kim. You have choices for this pregnancy."

Whoa. I cocked my head, unsure of what I'd heard. Choices? Oh, right—"choices."

Of course, he was telling me that if I didn't think I could handle a third child, because of the difficult road I faced with Mia and Gianna, I could terminate my pregnancy.

"No, Dr. P., I appreciate your concern and your medical information," (he was not pressuring or counseling me in any way, just informing me) "but I'll have this baby regardless of our circumstances with Mia and Gigi."

Bella bounced into the dining room as we were eating—the perfect exclamation point to my "so, Father, let me tell you about the day I was offered an abortion" story.

The good father smiled at Bella and said I had a beautiful pro-life story. And I suppose I do. I know of a woman who became pregnant with triplets via in vitro fertilization, but who aborted one of the fetuses, preferring to have only twins. That shocked me, and still does. But I know that there are instances when a woman might have to make the choice for less selfish reasons. I also know a certain mother who might have to make that choice for her daughters.

If Mia, Gianna, and/or Bella were, well, you know, imagine what could happen to a beautiful woman with a communication disorder—in the care of God knows who throughout her fertile years. I would not require my daughters to bear a child. I think the topic is supremely personal and unless faced with the choice, most women don't even know what they would do, despite what you might imagine beforehand. It's easy to say, "I'd never!" and I believe that never is best. But I don't live in a black-and-white world.

I feel the same way about vaccination. Every parent has to do their own homework and consult with their pediatrician to determine family history, possible allergies to ingredients (the flu vaccine is grown on a chicken egg), and other contraindications that might necessitate altering the pediatric vaccine schedule. Does that sound like crazy talk to you? I sure don't think so. How is "look before you leap" unsound advice?

Mainstream pediatricians have counseled parents on how to best alter the vaccine schedule to their children's needs. Dr. Bob Sears wrote a book called *The Vaccine Book* that helps parents to learn if, when, and how to revise the current vaccination schedule for their own child's health. He's hardly a zealot or fringe physician.

We've moved often enough that the girls have had at least five pediatricians since their autism diagnosis, and none has ever rejected us because of my views on vaccination. I always approach the topic from a position of informed choice and medical history. All three of my girls have autism and have had at least one seizure. Based on that information, I share that I am uncomfortable vaccinating Gianna and Mia beyond the shots they'd gotten from birth to ages three and four respectively and that I understand the gravity of my decision. I do everything but kneel down on the floor and beg for their forgiveness. A little humility goes a long way. My New York City cabdriver whose cab I took one day had a little sign on his glove box that read, A hostile attitude provokes a hostile response. I try to remember that phrase, and while I fail miserably at times, when it comes to my kids, I can bite my tongue.

When the H1N1 virus hit America in the spring of 2009, I was very concerned that this new virus could severely sicken my children—young children were thought to be the most vulnerable. I did not rule out the possibility of giving them the vaccination. I was genuinely concerned when the outbreak first hit our shores.

America's parents were exposed to a media frenzy of fear that suggested the flu would kill our kids. The vaccine hit the scene faster than McDonald's can pump out hamburgers. People who wouldn't buy an iPhone in its first model year rolled up their sleeves and their kids' sleeves, too.

We did not give the girls the H1N1 vaccination, nor (fortunately) did they become ill. I know several families whose kids were thought to have contracted the H1N1 flu (there was no formal testing), but they had mild to moderate symptoms and, fortunately, all recovered just fine.

My best friend in the world gave her daughter Gardasil (so much for my incredible negative influence on parents). I did not, having been contacted by numerous mothers whose daughters have had severe reactions, including death. Now young men are starting to feel the adverse side effects as this "cervical cancer" vaccine is re-marketed to boys, who, if you recall your seventh-grade health class, do not have cervixes.

What do you do if you don't feel it's safe to give your infant or child all of the vaccines at once but you still want the child to go to day care and then school? There are religious, philosophical, and medical exemptions that vary from state to state. My kids have been in public school in three states without being fully vaccinated for their age group, and with no problems. I agree that if there is an outbreak of an infectious disease, I will remove my children from school. Voilà. You can go to the National Vaccine Information Center (www.nvic.org) to find out the available exemptions in your state.

We have vaccine exemptions for a reason. Not every human on earth can handle every vaccine in existence without any risk of side effects. We've grown to think of vaccines as innocuous jabs that protect us without question. Criminy, you can get a flu jab at the Giant Eagle grocery store from a twelve-dollar-an-hour nurse's aide while you run in to pick up milk and bread. What happens if you have an adverse reaction at home? Are you going to scoot back into the store and ask the checkout clerk for help? The butcher? The baby formula and sinus medication are sold behind the counter, but vaccines are dosed like water.

It's something to think about.

Schools are paid per shot administered when they become vaccine clinics, too, and that especially galls me. A girl can't bring in a Midol pill for cramps without being suspended for a drug infraction, but a clinic can be set up in the cafeteria where kids are jabbed bing bang boom without Mom and Dad nearby. Again, what if there's an adverse reaction? A seizure or even just fainting? I think vaccines are best left to real doctors in offices where medical care is handy instead of being dosed willy-nilly around town.

I might as well get all the controversy out at once. Let's talk about mercury.

I don't believe it's wise to inject mercury into humans. And Thimerosal, the mercury-based medical preservative, is still in some vaccines given to children, despite the claims that it is not.

Seasonal flu, H1N1, and tetanus booster each contain twenty-five micrograms of mercury. There are pediatric versions of the flu shots, but they can be hard to find and are only recommended for children under age three. I'm not sure what happens to a kid at three that suddenly mercury is no longer dangerous. Mercury is also used in the manufacturing process of other vaccinations, and it is extracted to extremely low levels before the final product is complete. Some kids with peanut allergies go into anaphylaxis with just a sniff, so "extremely low" or "trace" levels of any potential allergen or neurotoxin isn't all that comforting to me.

For that reason, if anyone asked me about giving their child a flu shot, I would answer, "Well, there is mercury in the vaccine, and that troubles me. If your child has a preexisiting condition that makes flu a deadly threat, talk to your doctor about your options. I do not give my children seasonal or H1N1 vaccines."

And then I'd let the parent decide. That's called being pro–informed choice, not anti-vaccine. The person frequently blamed for starting the "anti-vaccine" movement is Dr. Andrew Wakefield, a gastroenterologist from England who touched off a decade-plus-long firestorm of controversy about the MMR (measles, mumps, rubella) vaccine.

In February 1998, The British Medical Journal *The Lancet* published a paper authored by Dr. Wakefield. His article suggested a *possible but yet unproven* connection between bowel disease and the MMR vaccine. His article focused on a case study of twelve children with neuropsychiatric disorders and bowel disease. At a press conference highlighting the release of his article, Dr. Wakefield suggested breaking up the Measles, Mumps, and Rubella (MMR) vaccine into three separate injections for safety reasons. After that suggestion, MMR vaccination rates dropped in Great Britain, causing great concern to public health officials.

Dr. Wakefield's original study never stated that the MMR vaccine caused autism. The following is taken straight from his original study:

We did not prove an association between measles, mumps, and rubella vaccine and the syndrome (autistic enterocolitis) described.

We have identified a chronic enterocolitis in children that may be related to neuropsychiatric dysfunction. In most cases, onset of symptoms was after measles, mumps, and rubella immunisation. Further investigations are needed to examine this syndrome and its possible relation to this vaccine.

Unfortunately for Dr. Wakefield, the MMR vaccine had been called into question just a few years earlier, when the mumps component was shown to cause febrile seizures in a small percentage of recipients. Ultimately, the formulation was changed to a different strain of mumps, and a new vaccine was released. Dr. Wakefield's paper raised further concerns among the already uneasy public. And the media, in an effort to protect the integrity of public health programs and corporate interests alike, pilloried Dr. Wakefield and his colleagues.

On January 28, 2010, Dr. Wakefield was found to have "failed in his duties as a responsible consultant" and went against the interests of children in his care in conducting research. On May 24, the General Medical Council revoked Dr. Wakefield's medical license, which in the UK is called "being erased from the medical register." It was a stunning, although not unexpected, blow:

Accordingly the Panel has determined that Dr. Wakefield's name should be erased from the medical register. The Panel concluded that it is the only sanction that is appropriate to protect patients and is in the wider public interest, including the maintenance of public trust and confidence in the profession and is proportionate to the serious and wide-ranging findings made against him.

The effect of the foregoing direction is that, unless Dr. Wakefield exercises his right of appeal, his name will be erased from the Medical

Register 28 days from when formal notice has been deemed to be served upon him by letter to his registered address.

Meanwhile, I can tell you that Dr. Wakefield appears at virtually every autism conference and speaks to parents about how they can address their children's terrible gut dysfunction. To some in the autism community, he is a hero and a martyr. To others, including the mainstream media, pharmaceutical companies, and public health officials (for whom vaccination is as much about sheer numbers and herd immunity as it is a medical procedure that affects individuals) he is a demon and scoundrel.

I highly recommend that you read his book *Callous Disregard* (which was the term the General Medical Council used to describe his work with children) and learn how his scientific studies led Dr. Wakefield into the snake pit that awaits vaccine questioners. You can draw your own conclusions about his work.

In a world where we mistrust pretty much every industry and corporation, including pharma, whose drugs are often recalled and given black-box warnings for their severe side effects, it strikes me as curious that the public is willing to assume that vaccines are safe for everyone at all times and that those of us who question their safety are the kooks.

It's the autism community that has been the most vocal about vaccine safety. So we're an easy target. The doctor leading the charge against the autism/vaccine safety community went so far as to write a book called *Autism's False Prophets* in which he "debunks" various treatments for the disorder. (I agree with him in some instances. Where there are desperate parents, abandoned by mainstream medicine, charlatans are sure to follow with miracle cures.) And then he launched an autism foundation to study (I kid you not) everything except vaccines as a potential trigger for autism. His name is Paul Offit.

Dr. Offit is coinventor of one of the more recent additions to the pediatric vaccine schedule. The vaccine is called RotaTeq from Merck. It makes sense that a vaccinologist and infectious disease expert would help create a new vaccine. There's nothing untoward about that at all. In the third world, rotavirus causes diarrhea and can be deadly. However, in America, with access to clean water, medical care, and electrolyte beverages, it's not a serious threat to our children's health. And yet it's on the American Academy of Pediatrics schedule in three orally administered doses.

Vaccines are big pharma business today. They keep pediatricians' offices busy (did your mom take you to the doctor for those nine "well" visits before the age of two?). The days of creating a medicine for the greater good are long gone. Jonas Salk, inventor of the polio vaccine, did not even patent his creation. From Wikipedia:

He had no desire to profit personally from the discovery, but merely wished to see the vaccine disseminated as widely as possible. When he was asked in a televised interview who owned the patent to the vaccine, Salk replied: "There is no patent. Could you patent the sun?"'

Today, it looks like you can patent the sun and then claim it doesn't cause skin cancer.

Here's part of the "Who We Are" from his organization, called Autism Science Foundation (www.autismsciencefoundation.org):

Vaccines save lives; they do not cause autism. Numerous studies have failed to show a causal link between vaccines and autism. Vaccine safety research should continue to be conducted by the public health system in order to ensure vaccine safety and maintain confidence in our national vaccine program, but further investment of limited autism research dollars is not warranted at this time.

However, in May 2008, Dr. Bernadine Healy, former head of the National Institutes of Health and the American Red Cross, made the bold statement that the vaccine autism link has not been "debunked," in a filmed interview with Sharyl Attkisson on CBS News:

Dr. Bernadine Healy is the former head of the National Institutes of Health, and the most well-known medical voice yet to break with her colleagues on the vaccine-autism question.

In an exclusive interview with CBS News, Healy said the question is still open.

"I think that the public health officials have been too quick to dismiss the hypothesis as irrational," Healy said.

"But public health officials have been saying they know, they've been implying to the public there's enough evidence and they know it's not causal," Attkisson said.

"I think you can't say that," Healy said. "You can't say that."

Healy goes on to say public health officials have intentionally avoided researching whether subsets of children are "susceptible" to vaccine side effects—afraid the answer will scare the public.

"You're saying that public health officials have turned their back on a viable area of research largely because they're afraid of what might be found?" Attkisson asked.

Healy said: "There is a completely expressed concern that they don't want to pursue a hypothesis because that hypothesis could be damaging to the public health community at large by scaring people . . . First of all," Healy said, "I think the public's smarter than that. The public values vaccines. But more importantly, I don't think you should ever turn your back on any scientific hypothesis because you're afraid of what it might show."

Upton Sinclair, who wrote *The Jungle* in 1906 about the meat-packing industry and the working class, said it best: "It is difficult to get a man to understand something when his salary depends upon his not understanding it."

Heck, cigarette manufacturers sat in front of Congress day after day declaring that their products did not cause cancer. Some probably even believed their own words. Doctors used to promote "healthy" cigarettes. Times change. Knowledge changes. And times are changing despite Dr. Offit's best efforts to scream like young Kevin Bacon in *Animal House, "All is calm!"* as the parade churned out of control before him.

All is not calm.

Educated, informed parents, most of whom are not in the autism world, are choosing to alter the pediatric vaccinations schedule, as reported by ABC News in May 2010:

> *The percentage of parents who refused or delayed vaccinations for their children rose sharply in the past decade, a study presented at a medical conference today showed.*
>
> *Refusal or delay of vaccines jumped from 22 to 39 percent between '03 and '08. Thirty-nine percent of parents refused or delayed vaccinations for their kids in 2008, up from 22 percent in 2003, according to the study by the Centers for Disease Control and Prevention, the University of Rochester, and the National Opinion Research Center.*
>
> *Parents refused or delayed vaccinations for various reasons, including the health of the child, the belief that recommended vaccines were excessive, questions about their effectiveness and concerns about possible side effects such as autism—although there's no scientific link.*

J. B. Handley, who continues to grace Age of Autism with his sharp wit and resourceful journalism, called The Children's Hospital of Philadelphia to see if he could secure an appointment with pediatrican Dr. Offit for "his child." He wrote about the call on October 26, 2009:

Given Offit's developing "expertise," I placed a phone call last week to his office in Philadelphia. While I knew the answer, it was still shocking to have the conversation, which went like this, with me ("JB") talking to Offit's assistant ("OA"):

JB: Hi, I have a child with autism, and I'd like to make an appointment to see Dr. Offit.

OA: He doesn't see patients.

JB: My son, he has autism, he needs help. My understanding is Dr. Offit is an expert on autism, he wrote a book, I'd really like to see him.

OA: He doesn't see patients in a clinical outpatient setting.

JB: Well, is there some other way for me to see him? Please, my son, he needs help, can't Dr. Offit make an exception?

OA: He doesn't see patients at all. I'm sorry.

Imagine if the dude who invented a new cigarette filter had written a book debunking lung cancer treatments and then gone on to found a group dedicated to finding the cause of lung cancer, and would look at everything except for cigarettes. Would your eyebrows be up around your hairline?

Unlike drugs, vaccines are exempt from medical liability, and have their own court system called the "Vaccine Court." If you or your child is injured by a drug or a physician's medical error, you can go to a trial by a jury of your peers. Not so with vaccines. You go before the Office of the Special Masters in a *no-fault* system that does not include a jury.

Vaccines are mandated for school attendance and in some instances, for employment. And when the government adds a vaccine to the pediatric schedule, it's a sales bonanza.

If ten people in California get sick from E. coli, the government seems to be able to track down the exact spinach plants responsible as well as the bird that flew overhead and pooped on them.

Tens of thousands of parents over the course of two decades have reported adverse reactions to vaccinations and a resultant autism diagnosis. And yet still we have no answers as to cause or prevention from the CDC. But "everyone knows" it's *not* vaccines.

Here's an excerpt about the vaccine market from an Associated Press article dated November 2009 that might help explain why vaccines are off the hook:

Vaccines are no longer a sleepy, low-profit niche in a booming drug industry. Today, they're starting to give ailing pharmaceutical makers a shot in the arm.

The lure of big profits, advances in technology, and growing government support has been drawing in new companies, from nascent biotechs to Johnson & Johnson. That means recent remarkable strides in overcoming dreaded diseases and annoying afflictions likely will continue.

"Even if a small portion of everything that's going on now is successful in the next ten years, you put that together with the last ten years (and) it's going to be characterized as a golden era," says Emilio Emini, Pfizer Inc.'s head of vaccine research.

Vaccines now are viewed as a crucial path to growth, as drugmakers look for ways to bolster slowing prescription medicine sales amid intensifying generic competition and government pressure to cut down prices under the federal health overhaul.

Unlike medicines that treat diseases, vaccines help prevent infections by revving up the body's natural immune defenses against invaders. They are made from viruses, bacteria, or parts of them that have been killed or weakened so they generally can't cause an infection.

Investment in partnerships and other deals to develop and manufacture vaccines has been on a tear—and accelerating since the swine flu pandemic began. Billions in government grants are bringing better, faster ways to develop and manufacture vaccines. Rising worldwide emphasis on preventive health care, plus the advent of the first ,.ultibillion-dollar vaccines, have further boosted their appeal.

While prescription drug sales are forecast to rise by a third in five years, vaccine sales should double, from $19 billion last year to $39 billion in 2013, according to market research firm Kalorama Information. That's five times the $8 billion in vaccine sales in 2004.

"What was essentially 25 years ago a rounding error now has become real money," says Robin Robertson, director of the U.S. Biomedical Advanced Research Development Authority.

That jump is due to a couple of new blockbuster vaccines and rising use of existing ones. The government's list of recommended vaccines for children since has more than doubled since 1985 to 17. It now also calls for a half-dozen vaccines for everyone over 18 and up to four more for some adults.

Parents of kids with autism are going broke. Doctors like Andrew Wakefield have spent their life's savings defending themselves against legal recrimination for having dared to even suggest that a vaccine could pose a problem. Meanwhile, school districts from Alaska to Maine are groaning under the weight of an ever-increasing enrollment of kids who need special education. And soon, that slew of kids born in the early 1990s, the leading edge of the epidemic, will be "aging out" of school by turning twenty-two. Is there a group home on your street yet?

Now, if Ebola comes to town, or anthrax or smallpox hits the air in a terror attack, I will be lined up to get my family vaccinated. I'm not stupid—contrary to what you'll read about me around the Internet.

As soon as medicine comes out with vaccines against some of the real threats my girls will face as women with autism—oh, things like physical and sexual abuse, employment discrimination, loneliness, housing crises—I'll roll up their sleeves myself.

MOTHER SUPERIOR

Oh, that Kim Stagliano has three, three(!) children with autism. I don't know how she does it!

★ ★ ★

If I had a nickel for every time I've heard those words from some well-intentioned mouth I'd have enough change to choke the CoinStar machine at the grocery store. (The CoinStar machine is a great way to entertain a child with autism, what with all the clinking and clanking and such. Sometimes you simply need to kill some time, what can I say?)

"How does she do it?" ranks right up there with "I'm sorry" in my lexicon of things people say to me or about me and my kids.

My usual answer is, "Well, they're kids, not appliances. They didn't come with guarantees, a warranty, or a return policy." It's a bit of a flippant response, but seems more motherly than, "I have no idea."

Was there some check-the-box quiz that I missed during pregnancy that would have ensured us three typical kids?

The fact is—what choice do I have? My girls have autism. Their father and I love them, and it is our duty and pleasure to care for them. Even when there's a whole lot of doody and very little pleasure.

Recently, however, at least two mothers on this planet decided they could no longer "do it," meaning care for their autistic child.

And so they murdered their severely autistic sons, each in a grue-some fashion.

The first story broke in New York City, as Gigi Jordan, referred to as a "socialite," although I don't know what that means circa 2010, stuffed her son full of pills while surrounded by luxury at the Peninsula Hotel in Manhattan.

The report in the *New York Daily News* read:

A multimillionaire mom fed her eight-year-old son a fatal dose of pills, then spent the night with his body inside a ritzy midtown hotel before a failed suicide try, police said.

Gigi Jordan was "babbling incoherently" after police kicked in the door of her $2,300-a-night suite at the Peninsula Hotel to find her son Jude faceup on the bed and foaming at the mouth, police sources said.

Jordan, 49, was surrounded Friday by hundreds of prescription drug pills and a rambling note expressing her love for the small boy who police say died at his mother's hands.

"I can tell you the only true happy moment in my life was when Jude was born," she wrote. "He was all the love I ever had in my life.

"He was the only thing that made me feel life was something of beauty, ever."

A police source said Jordan used a sofa to block the suite's bathroom door.

I'll give you a second to swallow the bile that just rose to your throat before telling you about the second murder, which took place in the United Kingdom. Ready? This report came from Damien Pearse of Sky News:

A mum has been charged with murdering her twelve-year-old autistic son by pouring bleach down his throat. The fourty-four-year-old woman, who has not been named, was arrested after police called at her home in Barking, East London.

The boy was taken by ambulance to hospital, but confirmed dead a short time later.

A post-mortem examination confirmed the cause of the boy's death as "ingestion of caustic liquid."

Police are investigating reports the dead child was given bleach after his mother said it was medicine.

The suspect was assessed by doctors before being handed back to police.

Neighbours said the boy was "severely autistic" and that his mother had been struggling to cope.

His eleven-year-old brother was placed in the care of social services.

Barking and Dagenham Council said: "This is a tragic incident. Our thoughts are with the family. A number of agencies have had involvement with them over several years, including the police, the NHS, and other local authorities.

"We are leading a serious case review as required by the Government to look into all details of this tragedy. A police inquiry is also currently under way."

Officers from the Metropolitan Police's Child Abuse Major Investigation Team are heading the inquiry.

The victim's mother will appear at Barking Magistrates Court this morning.

A distraught mother, at the end of her rope, poured bleach down her son's throat. That's not just murder. That's punishment, torture, the inflicting of intentional pain on her child. What dark hell was she in before commiting such an atrocity?

I wish I could tell you these murders are unusual. They are not. In 2006, a physician named Dr. Karen McCarron murdered her autistic three-year-old daughter. She put a plastic bag over her child's head and watched her suffocate to death. I Googled the question *how long does it take to suffocate?* and came up with anywhere from three to five minutes. I can't wait three minutes for water to boil on the stove.

Dr. McCarron held a bag tightly around her child's head for at least that. The child's name was Katie. Dr. McCarron is now serving a thirty-six-year sentence in an Illinois prison. As a physician, surely Dr. McCarron had access to a more human method to "euthanize" her child? It's the anger and brutality of the act that horrifies me almost as much as the killing itself.

I can't wrap my head around the cruelty of these murders. My maternal instinct rejects the notion entirely. And I abhor that these mothers can kill their children while sparing their own lives. Oh, Gigi Jordan "tried" to commit suicide but failed. She was a pharmaceutical executive who planned her son's murder by overdose carefully enough to book a luxury hotel room, to obtain and pack the pills (gee, do you use the Fendi valise or perhaps the Louis Vuitton?), and to then block the door with a sofa. Clearly she was sane enough to be able to think the murder through. So how come she's still alive?

Kids with autism are not without thoughts or feelings. Each child had to know what was happening to him or her. I'm sure they knew they were dying. It's almost too much for me to write the words.

Lest you think it's only the moms who crack, it happens to fathers too. In 2009, a father in Edmonton, Alberta, killed his eleven-year-old son and then committed suicide. Somehow, the suicide makes me feel a little better. Isn't that a sick admission? After reading that this boy had been in a group home and institutionalized, I can muster up a scintilla of empathy (not sympathy, there's a difference). From the CBC Web site:

The deaths of a man and his eleven-year-old autistic son on Sunday were the result of a murder-suicide, Edmonton police said Tuesday, after receiving confirmation from the Edmonton Medical Examiner's Office.

On Sunday, police found the bodies of the man, thirty-nine, and the boy in a home in northeast Edmonton, after they received a call from the man's common-law wife.

She was worried because she couldn't get in touch with him.

When officers arrived at the home around 12:42 PM, they found the man and the boy dead in the basement.

Police said they will not be releasing the names of deceased in order to protect the privacy of the family and to protect the identity of other children in the family. They will also not be releasing the cause of death.

The boy was autistic and had been living at a group home.

The family had become desperate for help because the little boy had become difficult for the family to manage, said Karen Phillips, who works with the Autism Society of Edmonton Area.

Phillips had worked with the family and said the mother asked her to share their story.

"The dad just felt he couldn't do it any longer and he just didn't think he could get the help he needed," she said, as her eyes welled up with tears.

At one point, the family took the boy to the emergency department of an Edmonton hospital, where he was later admitted to the psychiatric unit, Phillips said. But the staff there weren't equipped to help a child with autism.

Eventually, a place was found for the boy in a group home, but that search was a struggle, because many group homes are not set up to deal with autistic children with extreme behavourial problems.

The case highlights a lack of emergency services to help the families of autistic children, Phillips said.

"There is no emergency service. So parents are stuck at home with their children in situations that, if the general public knew, they'd be appalled," she said.

"They would think, 'None of us could cope with that.' But it's an everyday occurrence for families who have . . . behaviourally out-of-control children with autism."

Families are told to call police who in turn will take the child to the psychiatric unit of a hospital, but the staff there don't have the kind of training required to help the child, Phillips said.

"They're very good. They try their best, but they're not trained in autism and the doctors there will say clearly, this is not the place for children with autism."

The government was working on emergency respite services for families, but recent cutbacks mean the plans have been put on hold, she said.

The comment threads on the article are interesting. Most folks eviscerated Gigi Jordan, in part because of her wealth and the suggestion of mental instability over the years. The British mom was instantly branded a monster. However, some commenters with either an intimate or tangential link to autism talked about how they feel sympathy for each of these women or men, who were clearly deranged by their anger, loathing, grief, fear, frustration, exhaustion, loneliness, and the absolute drudgery of caring for an autistic child. My comment?

Fuck sympathy.

Yes, it's often sheer drudgery to care for an autistic child. From this I know. And I've felt every single one of those emotions in my years of caring for my daughters.

I've hauled one of my girls into the garage at three in the morning and put her into the minivan, shut and locked the doors while I walked back into the house to calm myself, get control of my anger, and escape the screaming fit that threatened to wake the entire house.

I've sobbed in a steaming hot shower to escape the smell of a crapisode and the resulting mountain of laundry waiting.

I've locked myself in my bedroom, sat on the edge of my bed, and lowered my head between my knees, willing myself to calm down while gasping for breath.

I sure as heck don't own a gun. Between my temper and Mark's, one of us would end up in a pine box.

The deaths of these children betray the growing tragedy that is autism. Yes, tragedy. Countless kids (literally countless, since the CDC can't seem to pinpoint exact numbers even as they can track down the single pig in Iowa that transmitted some rare disease) are suffering from autism, and so are their families. For most families, autism is a slog. It is 100 decathlons stacked on top of a thousand climbs to the top of Mt. Everest. You get to the top of the mountain and then another mountain appears in front of you. At the summit, when you die, is nothing but worry for the adult children you'll leave behind.

Bob Wright, cofounder of Autism Speaks, addressed the trauma on television a few years back, "Even if you're rich (which he is) autism leaves you broke." It sure can. Mark and I have learned that lesson all too well. We're digging out from a mountain of debt amassed courtesy of autism and unemployment.

I suppose that when you add the financial stress of autism to the emotional toll it takes, some folks will snap. Even people you'd expect to have their you-know-what together.

There was a wide-reaching controversy in the autism world in 2006, as Alison Tepper Singer, then Executive Director of Autism Speaks, made a startling admission in the documentary *Autism Every Day* by Lauren Thierry. She confessed that she'd thought about driving off of a bridge with her autistic daughter. A minority in the community voiced support for her honesty—that autism can indeed drive a parent to consider the unthinkable. Most felt the acknowledgment showed a stunning lack of hope and branded our children with autism as nothing more than a burden.

My children are not a burden. I carried them in my body and will carry them as long as they need me.

That doesn't make me a mother superior. Just a good mother.

BEEF: IT'S WHAT'S FOR BREAKFAST, LUNCH, AND DINNER

I first learned that diet could affect my kids when I met sarge Goodchild, a neurodevelopmental consultant in Massachusetts. He suggested that Gianna's red papery cheeks, runny nose, rheumy eyes, and less-than-angelic behaviors could be the result of consuming both wheat and dairy.

To tell you I was stunned is an understatement. Get rid of dairy? Never. Quit wheat? What on earth would they eat?

I'd fed my girls healthy foods since birth. I nursed Mia and Gianna for three and six months, respectively, and then I bought organic baby food and what I thought were healthy choices as they grew to be toddlers.

I reviewed Mia's eating habits. Eggo waffles, Annie's Macaroni and Cheese, goldfish crackers, pasta, and at least five or six sippy cups of milk per day. Uh-oh. Mia was on the white-foods-only autism diet track.

Of course, I didn't realize at the time that her eating habits could be indicative of a digestive problem related to her autism.

I ignored Sarge's advice for several months. Gianna's behavior worsened at preschool. She was bolting out of the classroom. Mia was becoming more lethargic and sluggish. Neither child was thriving.

With Sarge's help, I learned about the Defeat Autism Now! doctors who treat kids with autism. I booked an appointment in the spring of 2000.

Dr. Frank Waickman was about to retire. He had the kindly mien found in old-fashioned doctors. He was practicing for the love of his vocation, and it showed. He was the first doctor to ever ask me, "And how are you doing, Kim? How are you and your husband? Do you get out?" Mia and Gianna were young, and I was just starting to show with my pregnancy for Bella. I'll never forget that small bit of personal attention and kindness from him.

He tested the girls for food allergies (standard practice for many Defeat Autism Now! doctors) using sublingual (under-the-tongue) drops. If I hadn't seen the tests with my own two eyes, I'd never have believed any mom who told me that the tests could be so revealing. Remember, this was in 2000, long before I became an "anti-vaxxer crazy woman treating her kids with dangerous and untested products." Go ahead and roll your eyes with me, please? In fact, just three years earlier, I'd laughed out loud at a mom who was taking her son to a chiropractor for his ear infections. I was an allopathic-only idiot.

The girls were tested in a small room. The nurse placed three drops of a liquid under their tongues and waited for a reaction if there was one. I did not know what each test was for while the testing was in progress.

Within seconds of receiving the first drops, Mia's coloring went from straight lines to scribbles, then she dropped her crayon and slumped to the floor like a jellyfish. She was awake but completely stoned. I half expected her to demand a bag of Doritos and a cigarette. Antidote drops brought her back. That was her reaction to wheat.

Gianna had a series of drops that turned her into a fleeing, angry mess. She literally scaled over the children's gate to get out of the room. Her cheeks were flaming red, and she was belligerent. That was her reaction to dairy.

It was like the girls were puppets on strings and the various drops elicited a different performance. None terribly charming or worthy of an encore. I had to remove wheat and dairy from their diets.

Oh. My. God.

I have a cousin who developed or was diagnosed with celiac as an adult. Mark had had terrible digestive issues for much of his life, as had his siblings. And while I didn't have gastrointestinal (GI) problems, I was very much addicted to milk. As a small child I'd wake up in the night asking for milk. My parents joked that they'd considered putting a fridge on the second floor to save trips up and down the long staircase. I still love an ice-cold glass of milk before bed. I can feel myself calming down. The opiate effect. Gluten is the protein in wheat, rye, and barley. Casein is the protein in milk. People who have celiac disease cannot digest gluten. Those who are lactose intolerant and who avoid milk aren't necessarily intolerant of or allergic to milk protein. They are affected by lactose, which is milk sugar.

★ ★ ★

There's very little that's *free* about the gluten-free casein-free diet (GFCF). It's an expensive way to eat. Crummy, processed foods are always cheap. Adding healthier specialty foods to our diet meant shopping in mom-and-pop stores where the prices were sky-high. A big part of our autism expense was the girls' diet.

No matter what your food allergy or intolerance, the net result is *agita,* which is Italian for "pass the Alka Seltzer." And at first, the GFCF diet is a bellyache too. But not for long.

★ ★ ★

When I finally made the decision to go gluten-free and dairy-free, our first breakfast was orange juice and potato chips. I was lost. We began to eat an awful lot of meat. I knew that wasn't healthy for the girls.

So I started baking from scratch. I bought *Special Diets for Special Kids* by Lisa Lewis, PhD. That became my bible. I loaded up my pantry with weird flours and played crazy chemist daily. The kids adjusted really well. In fact, within the first week of dropping gluten, Mia ate a plate of veggies for the first time. We saw nothing but benefits from the diet. And continue to do so.

A favorite, kid-friendly meal is mock mac and cheese. I buy Trader Joes organic rice pasta and a bag of their frozen, organic mixed veggies and a box of Imagine-brand organic potato leek soup. Just boil the pasta until al dente (slightly undercooked for my non-Italian friends) and mix the soup, frozen veggies and pasta together in the pan after you've drained the macaroni. Pour the mixture into a greased casserole dish and top with the ultimate in comfort food toppings, crushed-up Ruffles potato chips. Bake at 350 degrees for about forty-five minutes. It feeds my three kids two hot meals, is cheap to make, and tastes good. Try it!

Today, there are dozens of great cookbooks, Web sites, and products dedicated to the GFCF diets. Companies have realized the size of the celiac and food intolerance market and responded to the demand with delicious, easy-to-use mixes and better labeling. In 2009, even Betty Crocker jumped on the gluten-free bandwagon with cake, cookie, and brownie mixes that are just delicious.

Simple substitutions, like using crushed rice cereal sprinkled with seasonings to make Italian breadcrumbs instead of a can of Progresso wheat-based crumbs, allow me to make cutlets and meatballs for the entire family.

There is emerging science about the GFCF diet for autism. Two studies came out concurrently last spring; one said there is a benefit, the other said there was not. It annoys me to no end that doctors who will prescribe a serious psychiatric drug to tamp down behavior will tell parents that the GFCF diet isn't safe or tested—"There's no science."

Are you kidding me? Tens of thousands of parents have seen results. Trust me, our kids aren't faking their tummy troubles. There's no placebo effect in autism. If your child suddenly stopped having daily acidic diarrhea that made his bottom bleed or BMs the size of a grapefruit that required an epidural to pass, would you say, "Aw, but there's no science, so I won't continue"? Not likely.

Have you got a beef with that?

YOU'VE GOT TO
FERTILIZE THE ROSES

In 2007, I coined a term that is now in the Urban Dictionary: the crapisode. It's not quite "Where's the beef?" or "Show me the money!" but it's my small contribution to the pop culture lexicon. I wrote a piece for The Huffington Post called, "The Crappy Life of the Autism Mom." If you've read this far into my book, you know that I do not genuinely believe that I have a crappy life. I'm pretty darn content overall and mostly cheerful, despite what the worry lines on my forehead tell you. My former career in advertising and promotions has taught me that headlines pull in readers. It doesn't matter if the headline intrigues or infuriates, the point is to grab attention when the reader has dozens of story choices on his or her screen at the moment. It's all about the clicks. If no one reads my posts, they can be as finely written as Shakespeare's plays, and I'll have accomplished much ado about nothing.

Bowel movements (BMs). Poop. Crap. The process of elimination has taken up an inordinate amount of my mothering skills thanks to autism. All parents have to deal with toilet training. And while the average age of having a fully trained child is creeping upward (Pampers came out with size-six diapers many years ago, and Pull Ups may soon be adding Penthouse Pet designs to their Dora the Explorer and Go, Diego, Go offerings), most families achieve the goal long before kindergarten.

Not us. Not most families in the autism world. Toilet training can be one of the toughest challenges when you have a child on the spectrum, with kids remaining in Pull Ups or adult diapers well into their elementary school years and beyond. Often the children have sensory issues that can impede their ability to feel when they have to pee or poop.

I started toilet training Mia and Gianna when they were three and four years old. I optimistically bought a book called *Toilet Training in Less Than a Day,* which, after two weeks of mopping up puddles on my floor, I renamed *Big Fat Crock of You Know What.*

I had charts, rewards, potty seats, a teddy bear that sung "I'm Super Duper Pooper," an Elmo doll that could pee in the toilet, and several books. One was called *Toilet Training for Individuals with Autism,* by Maria Wheeler, who explains in her introduction how difficult it is to train this population. I got nowhere with the girls using her technique and became so frustrated that I tracked down Maria Wheeler herself and begged her to come to Cleveland to train the girls. Mark and I spent hundreds of dollars with a psychologist to try and get them trained. All she did was sit them on a potty seat and have them push the button on a kiddie book that made a flushing sound. Man, those PhDs come in handy, don't they?

Gianna was finally trained by Mrs. D., the paraprofessional in her preschool. She sat Gianna down, ignored her frantic little screams of protest, and waited the child out. Plink plink poop! Once Gianna had gone a couple of times, she was on her own. She got it!

Mia took a bit longer—Mark and I used to joke morbidly that we'd be changing period pads and poop at the same time. It wasn't quite so funny when it came true. But Mia also mastered her bathroom skills. You'd think my experience would have made training Bella easier. Not at all. Because as the saying goes, "If you've met one person with autism, you've met one person with autism." Bella responded beautifully to a program I learned from a dynamo of a woman named Brenda Batts out of Dallas who I talked to at the National Autism Association Conference. She recently published *Ready, Set, Potty!* I was skeptical of her suggestions, the first of which required me to find silky panties for Bella. "What? Silky panties for my baby? Is Victoria's Secret that she pees in her pants?" Two and a half years after we tried Brenda's program, Bella is moving away from a toilet schedule where we take her every couple of hours to independence, where she seeks out the bathroom on her own.

Sometimes the poop is merely the medium. I know families whose kids smear theirs on the walls. One amazing dad created a "poop suit" for his teen son to wear to bed so that he could not have a BM at night and then destroy, er, *decorate* his bedroom, leaving his parents to attempt a daily cleaning ritual worthy of an operating room. I get e-mails from moms explaining that they put their son's pjs on backward so he can't work the zipper. Their Van Gogh brown period is not malicious, at least I don't think so. When we've had poop issues, they've usually been a result of one of our daughters wanting to change herself. In some ways, taking a blob of *you-know-what* out of the pants is progress. It means she's aware she has soiled her pants and wants relief. Okay, so that usually happens with a neurotypical kid when they're around two years old. It's funky when your child is eight or ten or twelve. But with autism, beggars can't be choosers, and when it happens in our household, I always try to chalk it up to forward movement, if you'll pardon a bad pun.

We had a "Mommy, I kinda sorta changed myself" incident a while back that made me laugh, cry, and then laugh again. One of the girls changed herself in her room. That means the pants come down and whatever is in them comes out, got it? Thanks to lots of bananas and proper nutrition, the movement is usually intact. As I walked upstairs, I smelled a little something that was more "oh my God" than eau-de-cologne.

Sure enough, there had been a *self-care* event. I cleaned up the situation and steam-cleaned the bedroom carpet. Honestly, given the ever-rising autism rates, consider giving a steam cleaner as a wedding gift, as chances are the bride and groom will need it when the kids come along. I checked under the bed and the baseboard heating units, around the closet, anywhere that things could have rolled. All clear.

The next day, I noticed "that smell" in the room. I did a poop check. Nothing. I took the laundry downstairs, thinking maybe that's what I was smelling.

Nope.

The next day, I did another poop check. Still nothing. I looked at the ceiling, just in case. I washed the sheets and comforter.

Nope.

The next day, I noticed something.

There, on the *Sesame Street* kitchen (remember the one that got trashed in the flood? I found it on sale that Christmas Eve and bought it) next to the closet, was a stove knob with Ernie's photo on it. Twist the knob and Ernie hollers, "Turn it up!" There, on the *Sesame Street* kitchen was a stove knob with Bert's photo on it. Twist it and Bert hollers, "Turn it down!" And there, between the two stove knobs, was a giant piece of old, dried-out poop. "Get the Lysol!" I screamed. I snapped a photo with my cell phone just to prove it had happened.

★ ★ ★

Poop is a real issue in the autism world, though one you don't often hear about. I don't mind talking about yucky. I wrote "The Crappy Life of the Autism Mom" to accomplish two goals. One, to show how different life is inside an autism household. And two, to explain to the non-autism world how I felt about a trend toward not respecting the needs of parents to treat their children's autism courtesy of the "neurodiversity" community. Neurodiversity can mean simple acceptance of different ways of thinking. And that's a great message. I want my kids to be accepted. Kind of a no-brainer, right? However, the message was hijacked by angry parents who've given up on their kids or who never had hope to begin with, medical skeptics with more time on their hands than compassion, and even high-functioning people with Asperger's or autism who advocate against treatment, hope, and recovery. Most of the negative Google alerts on my name come from the hardcore ND world.

Sometimes you have to stir the pot up a bit to make people outside the autism universe know just how absurd our lives are thanks to the nitwits who preach against helping our kids. Here's "The Crappy Life of the Autism Mom."

Well, that should set off alarm bells in the neurodiversity world.

Autism is like a box of Bertie Bott's Every Flavor Beans (from the Harry Potter books). Some autistics got the raspberry cream or root beer flavor. They can speak eloquently, write blogs, move out on their own, marry, have children, and manage their autistic traits. Others with autism, like my three girls, got the ear wax/vomit/dog poop flavor. They need help 24/7 to navigate the world. When I talk about autism, I mean the version that my three girls have. I'm not talking about the sort of autism that encompasses quirky kids with some social deficits who are otherwise brilliant.

The ND community tells me and tens of thousands of other parents that we are disrespecting our kids by trying to help them. The ND blogs berate us as wanting to change our kids because we don't accept them. Here's a "taste" of what autism looks like in the Stagliano household. Would you want something better for your kids?

Twice last month, we had a "crapisode." What is a crapisode? (This is where you might want to stop eating and put down your beverage.) My ten-year-old (No. 2, appropriately, for the purposes of this entry) pooped in the toilet. That is reason to cheer, believe me. Toilet training is a major issue in my section of the autism community. Our kids can wear diapers into their teens and beyond. So Miss G. pooped. Hooray! But Miss G. forgets to flush. And she rarely closes the lid. Not hooray.

Miss Peanut, my six-year-old, seems to believe that being a Virgo means she simply MUST swim in any puddle larger than spit. The toilet is like an Olympic-sized pool to her. So Peanut goes into the toilet after Miss G. has had her, ah, success. Peanut flings kaka everywhere and gets it all over herself, the floor, the walls, the tub, the baseboards, and the window. Wes Craven could not film anything scarier than what I saw that school morning, thirty-five minutes before the bus was due to arrive. That's a "crapisode." It happens in the blink of an eye while I'm washing dishes or doing laundry. I'm alerted by a splashing sound that drops a brick into my stomach. Miss G. doesn't understand to flush and close the lid. Miss Peanut doesn't realize that a face full of feces is rarely considered a way to amuse oneself outside the fetish community.

I will never stop trying to help my girls recover from their autism. I cannot tell you what recovery means. It varies by kid and according to God's grace. If recovery means only that Peanut understands she should sit on the toilet, not play in the toilet, I'll take it.

Recovering your kids doesn't mean denying their value as people. To the contrary, it means we are willing to devote our lives, our savings, our sanity to their improved health, development, and well-being.

Maybe we need an expanded vocabulary. The NDs can keep the word "autism," and my kids get a new label. Fine by me. Just don't tell me to give up on my girls and accept their version of autism (remember the Bertie Bott's beans) as simply a different type of personality. Because THAT'S a load of crap.

Published on HuffingtonPost.com, January 3, 2007.

★ ★ ★

The piece has traveled farther and wider than I ever get to go. Then again, I'm an autism mom times three, so I don't get out much. "Crappy Life" has been picked apart and scrutinized more than a specimen in a Great Plains Laboratory comprehensive stool analysis test.

With "Crappy Life" I did what many writers strive for—I struck a nerve. Many parents have thanked me for sharing the difficulties of trying to help a child with autism navigate day-to-day life. Others have berated me for embarrassing my children. Please. Embarrassment is my birthright. Ask anyone in my family about the little gifts my Grandma Yoli had to deal with after my diaper pooped out (literally) at the Farmer's Daughter gift barn in St. Johnsbury, Vermont, in the mid-sixties. They still tease me about "losing my marbles in Vermont" four decades later. The day my kids can read my writing and complain to me that I hurt their feelings will be the proudest day of my life. I will apologize to them and hope they understand that I was fighting for them through my words.

★ ★ ★   `

The neurodiversity situation shines a light on the fact that autism, as a spectrum disorder, has numerous "factions" for lack of a better word. Autism can look very different from one person to the next. Even my three girls present differently from each other, though each has an autism diagnosis. And the mainstream media, which is so adept at telling you when Brad Pitt has gone pee without getting Angelina's blessing, is woefully ignorant about autism. They use autism and Asperger's interchangeably, for instance. The two diagnoses are not the same, and there's much debate about that.

In 2010, the debate got more heated. There's a book published by the American Psychiatry Association (a.k.a. A Pill for All) called the *Diagnostic and Statistical Manual of Mental Disorders*. Yes, mental disorders. Autism is in there as a diagnosis. I do not think my kids are mentally ill for one minute. I think they have some sort of brain injury or difference that was created in them and that has upset, tipped over, and crushed the apple cart of their neurology.

In the fifth edition of *DSM-V* (yes, the Roman Numerals are to make the psychiatrists look much smarter than the rest of us) Asperger's will lose its own diagnosis code and become part of the autism code.

What does this mean?

A lot of folks in the Asperger's world do not care to be lumped into the autism spectrum. They do not relate to the challenges of full-blown autism. I can certainly respect that they do not want to be included in a group that includes the mentally challenged, or as I have read, "adults in diapers." Ouch.

Meanwhile, many parents of children and young adults with Asperger's support the revised definition since, traditionally, services and school support have been far lower for kids with Asperger's. Their impairments are not as glaring as a lack of speech. They can do the schoolwork, so they don't get services. They often falter socially and academically.

Asperger's is not without its own major challenges. While Aspergians are often thought of as occupying the "top" of some kind of pyramid scale, there are a lot of families with kids whose lives are very difficult because of Asperger's. I met a woman at church whose thirty-year-old cannot find a job. A good friend worries her son will threaten to bring a knife to school and be expelled. Asperger's is not Autism Lite.

The at-a-glance difference between an Asperger's diagnosis and autism is the communication deficit. Asperger's kids can speak, in fact are often hyperverbal, but are lacking in the social skills most of us take for granted, like being able to read emotions in faces, or understanding when a conversation has steered elsewhere and being able to adapt.

There is good news on the horizon for everyone with autism. After starting a chapter with poop, I want to finish up with the fresh scent of a rose. And thanks to John Robison, I can do that.

There is a study underway at Beth Israel Deaconess Hospital and Harvard Medical School in which people with Asperger's (like my friend and author John Robison, the first test subject) are altering the plasticity of their brains and ameliorating the negative symptoms of their Asperger's. That's a hoity-toity way of saying, "They are getting better!" This therapy is called TMS, short for Transcranial Magnetic Stimulation, and is part of a major study at Harvard under Dr. Alvaro Pascual Leone.

Here's a description of the therapy from the Berenson-Allen Center for Non-Invasive Brain Stimulation in Boston:

Transcranial magnetic stimulation or TMS is a neuro-physiological technique that allows the induction of a current in the brain using a magnetic field to pass the scalp and the skull safely and painlessly. In TMS, a current passes through a coil of copper wire that is encased in plastic and held over the subject's head. This coil resembles a paddle or a large spoon and is held in place either by the investigator or by a mechanical fixation device similar to a microphone pole. As the current passes through the coil, it generates a magnetic field that can penetrate the subject's scalp and skull, and in turn induce a current in the subject's brain. TMS is used in clinical neurophysiology to study the nerve fibers that carry the information about movements from the brain cortex to the spinal cord and the muscles.

Repetitive TMS (rTMS) can be used to study how the brain organizes different functions such as language, memory, vision, or attention. In addition, rTMS seems capable of changing the activity in a brain area, even beyond the duration of the rTMS application itself. In other words, it seems possible to make a given brain area work more or less for a period of minutes, or even weeks when rTMS is applied repeatedly several days in a row. This has opened up the possibility of using rTMS for therapy of some illnesses in neurology, rehabilitation, and psychiatry.

John Elder Robison also writes about TMS on his blog, which I suggest you read to learn more. In it he says, "*Shirley and Alvaro developed a theory that some parts of the autistic mind are overactive, and those overactive parts sort of overwhelm the other parts. By 'slowing down' the over-active areas they hoped to bring about an improvement in overall function.*"

Imagine not being able to read facial expressions and how tough that would make your life. Like if Jane at work is terribly sad and instead of acknowledging her teary eyes and quivering lips, you were to say, "Isn't the sunshine beautiful today, Jane?" She might think you were a jerk. You are not a jerk, but you cannot read her expression, so you say the wrong thing. And this happens to you over and over and over so that your life becomes a never-ending chain of social gaffes and failures, right from childhood. That's how John describes Asperger's. That's hardly Autism Lite.

My phone rang during the spring of 2008. It was John Robison. John isn't one to pick up the phone for chitchatty girl talk, as you can imagine. I'd never heard him so animated, and I'll not soon forget what he told me about his first changes from the TMS therapy trial, "Kim! I can read people's minds!"

Being a neurotypical female, my first thought was, "You can work for the psychic hotline and make a fortune!" This is not what John meant by reading minds. He meant that for the first time in his life, he understood emotions via facial expressions. Just imagine the veil of uncertainty that lifted for him. Jane wouldn't think he was a jerk, because he'd know to cluck cluck and maybe even pat her shoulder, rather than expound upon the lovely day.

As the months progressed and he continued the therapy, he experienced a number of positive changes: *"I can sum up what's it's done for me very succinctly. TMS has been the lever that allowed me to roll the boulder of autistic social disability out of my path. Today, thanks to Alvaro and his team, my world is brighter, more colorful, and more alive than anything I knew before. And best of all, I am fully engaged. I'm no longer an outsider. I have gone from feeling like a social outcast to feeling like I can talk to anyone, most any time. It's a magical thing."* John has tracked his progress with great honesty on his blog and continues to do so.

"Let me know when my girls can participate," I told him from the first time I heard about the therapy. TMS is noninvasive and all one has to do is sit there. I want to try every possible therapy I can for my kids. This one is particularly appealing because of the safety net of Harvard and John's assurances. I was born at Beth Israel in Boston. It would be pretty cool to get help for my kids there.

So a couple of nights ago, my phone rang during dinner. It was John. Again, he was not calling for girl talk. "Kim, the TMS therapy is going so well for Aspergians that we're going to begin trying it on lower-functioning kids. We've been able to affect speech, to bring it out. Your oldest daughter can participate." (Fifteen is the youngest age they will accept right now for ethical reasons.)

When the study starts, my Mia Noel will be on the list of subjects. We might be able to tweak her brain and help get rid of one of the most insidious aspects of her autism.

My Mia might speak.

Holy crap.

MY TURN

Most of my newer friendships have been born out of the shared experience of having a child with autism. Jane Doe will hear that Sally Smith is moving to town and send me an e-mail, "Hey, this mom has a son with autism. You should call her."

I usually make the call, because autism can make for an isolated life for us parents. I know I hate feeling alone. Although the Internet is a great connector, it's not a replacement for genuine friendship, despite the thousands of friends and followers you might have on Facebook or Twitter.

One of these friendships started several years ago, while we lived in Hudson.

I got a call that a woman named Sheila was moving to town with her teenaged daughter and husband in the hope of finding better schooling for her child.

Sheila had her hands full with her daughter, who had numerous diagnoses, one of which was autism. Sheila was a fantastic advocate for her daughter, and she pushed our school district to its limits, finally getting better programming than most of us ever imagined, including ABA therapy managed by the Cleveland Clinic school. At the same time, her husband's family-owned retail store was struggling. She and I were like two peas in a pod, sharing child issues and financial worries. I won't say misery loves company, because I've never been truly miserable with my life. But we did have a unique bond because of our circumstances.

One day, Sheila and I were having coffee and she asked a question that blew me away: "When is it going to be my turn?"

The years of caring for her aging parents and tending to her daughter had taken their toll. She was over fifty and perhaps the retrospection that comes with age brought her life into sharp focus. I was busy with a newborn, hadn't hit forty, and still had the doe-eyed hope that I'd "fix" my kids in a couple of years and then get on with my life. Hardy har har.

Here I am, many years after she asked me that unanswerable question. My kids still struggle mightily. We've been through three bouts of unemployment. Our last three homes have been little more than bivouacs as we've traipsed about New England.

And yet I have never once asked, "When is it my turn?"

This *is* my turn.

I love my life. That doesn't mean I wouldn't change the autism part for the girls. If I had a magic wand I'd wipe the autism right out of their lives like peeling off the skin of an orange. I know there is sweet fruit hidden under the bitter pith and the rough skin.

How many people can honestly say they wouldn't change anything about their lives?

Have you ever sat in church and prayed for something very specific? I didn't used to. It seemed presumptuous to make demands of God. I preferred to do what most women do—assume our men are telepathic and that they understand a quick snort of breath is actually our way of saying, "Could you please take out the trash?" I'm guilty of that every day. Poor Mark! My language is different from his. He's direct and I'm oblique.

One Sunday during Mass, our pastor said something that struck me during the homily. (Yes, Father, I do pay attention!) He told us we have to be very specific in our prayers to God. I was taken aback. It feels supremely presumptuous, to talk to God like I'm ordering from a takeout menu.

"Yeah, God? Gimme a No. 7, the executive job for my husband with a supersized salary, and a side order of cure for my kids' autism." I can feel the earth opening up and swallowing me whole just thinking that directly in terms of prayer. And yet, I'm learning to do just that. And (wait, let me toss salt over my shoulder here to ward off the devil) it's working.

I used to pray big thoughts like, "Please let me get married," when I was dating my high school sweetheart. I didn't mention the potential groom by name because I assumed that God knew who I meant.

God sure knew better than I did.

At the risk of sounding like a slogan on a bumper sticker, I know that I am not living in some sort of dress rehearsal. It's showtime every morning I wake up. Some days I'm living in a comedy, others a tragedy, and once in a blue moon, a romance. I just can't think of myself on "hold" until some sweeping change affects me.

I've wondered what kind of mom I'd have been if my girls had the luxury of being neurotypical. With my pushy personality, maybe I'd have become an intolerable stage mother, pushing a breathtaking toddler named Mia into dancing school recitals. I could have been a soccer team sideliner screaming at Gianna to run faster, to score more goals, and to tug the hair of the defense person covering her. Maybe I'd have Bella at the skating rink at five in the morning seven days a week practicing her figure eights and jumps until her bottom was bruised from the falls.

I'll never know.

And I don't much care.

Don't misunderstand me, I'd love to worry to death about sixteen-year-old Mia on her first date with a boy I thought was too mature for her. It would be sublime to hear Gianna tell me she hates me and slam her door in a fourteen-year-old's classic huff. If only Bella could roll her eyes at me in disgust for reminding her to brush her teeth for the umpteenth time—instead of having to brush her teeth myself.

Sometimes I have to fight the pain of going down the "what if . . ." path. If I start thinking about all of the losses the kids experience—and Mark and me, too—my breathing gets too shallow to be healthy. My heart beats too fast. I have to remind myself: This *is* my turn.

I get reminders every day of the differences in my kids. Every afternoon, Bella returns from school on a small school bus. The driver's daughter, just two years old, rides along in her car seat. The other day, she looked right at me, waved and said, "Hi!" My own daughter was staring out the window. Yes, that hurts.

★ ★ ★

On the flip side, Mark and I have the great honor of tiny, sometimes daily moments of heroics in the girls. When you're truly hungry, a simple meal is as good as a feast. The other day, Mia awoke and told me, "Tuesday. Swimming." It reminds me that even in her relative silence, Mia is aware of her world and engaged in school. I felt proud of her.

Gianna has always had a lovey she carried. As a toddler it was a teddy bear that somehow got lost between Pennsylvania and Ohio. She had her blankey for many years until it wore down to mere scraps (that I've saved). In Ohio, we had a carbon monoxide scare, and she was given her manatee plush toy by the responding firefighter. Manatee was by her side for four years. I had to perform countless surgeries on the poor thing as he continued to fall apart. In sixth grade she read a picture book about emotions called *The Way I Feel*, and connected (that's a kinder way of saying became obsessed) with the page that described the feeling "excited." Despite my limited sewing skills, I was able to create a Halloween costume for her and she became "Excited" straight from the book. She was thrilled.

She lost interest in Manatee (don't tell her, but he's hidden in my closet) and started carrying that book around every waking minute for close to two years. She even slept on it. It fell apart despite yards of clear tape covering the spine and curling pages, and Mark would always order another copy online. We might be responsible for its latest printing.

We took a family photo during the 2009 holidays, and I'm proud to say *The Way I Feel* has been replaced with a photocopy of our family photo. Gianna carries it everywhere (except school) and sleeps with it covering her face. It's a form of autistic perseveration, I realize that. But it's important to her and fills a need. I can't deny her that. That the loveys have evolved from a toddler's toy to a family photo shows emotional growth. I'm proud of Gianna.

Bella, my quiet one, delights us in her own way. One night, after years of tucking her in, kissing her forehead, and waving good-bye as I closed her door, she looked right at me and waved back! She waved back! Tears came to my eyes. (Darn it, even now my screen is getting blurry as I write this, remembering her very real communication.)

Mark and I take nothing for granted. It's an intense, emotional, joyful way to live, even if the big picture sometimes looks bleak. I like it.

God's plan for our financial picture has also been so different from what I'd expected. Please, we're the coiners of the "Stagtastrophe," why would I ever have thought it would be otherwise?

I married in part for corporate security. At the end of my dad's career as an orthodontist, there was no gold watch, no pension, no 401(k), no retirement benefits beyond social security and Medicare. I craved the safety and buttoned-down conformity of the corporate life. I married a corporate man with a corporate father.

Nineteen years and seven jobs later, five of which ended not by choice, my husband is now self-employed. He runs the Stagliano Group, and is an independent sales rep for a handpicked selection of vendors. He has created a pot of gold. Gold smells a lot better than the chamber pots we'd been clawing out of for so long. He said to me one day with a wicked grin, "This is like having a license to print money." God knows we need plenty of it to get out of debt and squirrel away a fortune for the girls.

He's a success because he's respected and trusted. His company is growing every day. There's now money in my bank account on the thirty-first of the month. (Where's that saltshaker? I feel jinxed even mentioning Mark's success.)

As our married life and our financial life become more stable, I feel hopeful that my sometimes paralyzing fears about the girls' futures will subside as we help them build happy, safe, adult lives. Will they live under our roof until we're old? Will they find a shared community home with support?

I don't know.

But I'm learning to trust in God that I'll find the right answers because God *has* answered many of my prayers.

This *is* my turn.

I'm not going to waste it.

AUTHOR'S NOTE

In the spring of 2010, a trinity of events took place that squired my family through most of the Trumbull Police Department. On March 1, I was seated at my desk in my home office when I heard the sound of breaking glass.

I stood, startled, and quietly moved toward the front kitchen window and peered into the driveway.

There was a dark green sedan backed up to my garage door.

Holy sh★t, someone is invading the house.

My guardian angel, or maybe my reptilian brain, took over. We have very poor cell phone reception in our neighborhood so I grabbed the portable phone off the kitchen counter and hightailed it out my front door, just as the marauders (how often do you get to use that in context?) snuck in the garage entrance just behind the desk where I'd been working seconds ago.

I crouched down under the bushes in my front yard and called 911.

"I'm being robbed!"

I was shaking, staring back at my own house, wondering what was happening inside. I knew it wasn't a tea party.

Within ninety seconds a cruiser pulled across my driveway. I pointed toward the garage. The policeman drew his gun and entered the house.

Moments later two men burst out of my front door wearing ski masks. One ran across the street, the other tried to steal the police car. It was locked, so he ran across the street, too. They disappeared into the narrow riverbed that winds through our neighborhood.

Long story short, the police caught one guy and he is now in prison. The other was never found. The car they left in my driveway was loaded with loot (again, who uses that word for real?). Mark and I lost a few pieces of valuable jewelry that were never recovered, but I was safe.

The local paper proclaimed, Mom of Three Busts Crime Ring! I even reenacted my part in the drama on the local Fox news channel.

That's how we met the detective in the Robbery Division.

In June, Bella and I were driving home from a trip to the bank on a clear Friday evening when our car was rear-ended, giving both of us whiplash. An eighteen-year-old had taken his eyes off the road and slammed into us. Poor Bella was scared to death. I was mostly pissed off.

That's how we met the officers in the Traffic Division.

The third contact with the police is hard to talk about. It's harder to put it onto paper.

In 2010, Bella presented four different times with an ugly, black-and-blue bruise on the top of her hand, between her thumb and Mr. Pointer. I took Bella to the pediatrician. We got X-rays. We tested for a clotting disorder. The injury was a mystery. Neither her teachers nor I could recall any incident that would create such havoc on her hand. Then, a friend who is a sports physical therapist examined the last of the four injuries and told us it was a sprain. The kind of injury that requires real force.

Through a process of elimination, we determined the one place it could be happening. We were able to watch audio/video tapes that showed an adult making contact with Bella, and we could hear Bella screaming, her body obscured behind her abuser.

There was a series of attacks over the course of two months, all recorded on security tapes.

Watching those tapes made me sick to my stomach. When Mark saw them, he said very quietly, "I've never felt such rage in my life."

That's how we met the detective in the Juvenile Division.

Bella does not speak—yet. She weighs sixty-three pounds soaking wet. She is passive.

She is my baby.

Her abuse is another reason I will never stop fighting for research into autism's cause, for better treatments, and for therapy, and very soon I'll be focusing on adult issues with the same intensity.

I'm no Mother Teresa. But I am a Mother Warrior.

Take care.

Kim

ENCORE

Having read about our police interaction has likely left you fuming and more than a little curious. Unlike my hardcover readers, who were left hanging, you, my paperback friends, get the full story right now. Yay for immediate gratification! Booooooo for the actual story. Here goes.

In March of 2010, Bella, our youngest, came home from school with an ugly purple bruise on the fleshy part of her hand between her pointer finger and her thumb. It was swollen and clearly painful to the touch. School sent home a note in our communication log, "Did Bella hurt herself at home?" I wracked my brain trying to recall if she'd fallen or done anything to cause this mystery bruise. I called our pediatrician to report the injury and was told to apply the usual treatment of a cold compress, watch for swelling, maybe some Motrin. Fine.

Except all was not fine. This bruising happened again. And again. And both school and I started to worry big time that this wasn't an accidental injury. I was sick. And scared. And pissed.

I was standing in the post office in May when my phone rang. "Kim, it's the school nurse. Bella has another bruise starting and she came off the school bus in hysterics—crying, agitated, upset."

The school bus? With the nice driver and her daughter the bus monitor, a kid of twenty-four who had brought her own babies onto the bus many times? We'd known them for over a year. I'd cootchie-cooed the baby. Was this bus monitor hurting my child?

The next school day, a team including Mark and me, Bella's teacher, the SPED director, principal of her school, and director of transportation watched the school bus security tape. Each of us turned a shade of angry red or in my case "about to pass out white." There on tape we saw the monitor stand up, leave her seat, move back to sit across the aisle from my (quiet) Bella, reach across into Bella's seat with her arms ... and suddenly you hear Bella *cry out in pain*!

We sat in stunned silence. Mark said later, "I've never felt such rage in my life."

From there, the system took over. School called Child Services and the police. Within an hour we had an officer in our home taking a statement. The detective assigned to the case, Kevin Hammel, reviewed every minute of bus tape available, putting together a case against the bus monitor, Jennifer Davila. She was arrested in August of 2010, and charged with three counts of Risk of Injury to a Minor and three counts of Assault on a Handicapped Person.

Davila pleaded guilty under the Alford Doctrine to second-degree Reckless Endangerment and was sentenced by Superior Court Judge Frank Iannotti to a suspended six-month term and eighteen months probation.

But the story didn't end there. Come on, we're the Staglianos, coiners of the word Stagtastrophe! While reviewing the bus tapes, Detective Hammel noticed that the driver, named Evelyn Guzman, and also Jennifer Davila's *mother*, was sending and receiving text messages while operating a school bus! This was news to Mark and me and the other parents of the kids who rode that bus. We never saw her holding a cell phone. She was smart enough to hide it from the parents.

Verizon phone records showed 1068 messages sent in a brief time period. Can you imagine the audacity, the disregard for safety (her own daughter and grandchildren rode the bus!) and the pure hubris of Guzman? Neither could the detective. You should not piss off a tall, beefy detective with a cold hard gun on his hip and a soft spot for kids. In March 2011, he had her arrested and charged with Risk of Injury to a Minor and Reckless Endangerment. The arrest made the national news.

Because Guzman was a first time offender, she was eligible for a Connecticut program called accelerated rehabilitation (AR). If granted by the judge, she would face some penalties but have a *clean record* after two years. *Are you kidding?* When a defendant applies for AR, the victim(s) or family receives a letter from the defense attorney stating we had the right to protest in front of the judge.

Do you think I protested?

I started an online petition, gathered 1099 names from around the globe, from every corner of the autism community, and in a week's time Mark and I showed up at the courthouse with over eighty pages of petition signatures printed out onto a sheaf of pink paper. Bella's photo was on the cover sheet. Several parents of other children who rode the bus also attended the court hearing. Here is the statement I read in a clear voice, trying to read and glance up to make eye contact with the judge as many times as possible:

Good morning, Your Honor. And thank you for this opportunity. My name is Kim Stagliano. My husband Mark and I have three daughters with autism. Our youngest, Isabella, rode Evelyn Guzman's elementary school special education bus. Last week, Ms. Guzman's daughter Jennifer Davila pleaded guilty under the Alford Doctrine to second-degree reckless endangerment after having been arrested for assaulting Bella numerous times on the school bus. It was the video tape review for that case that led Detective Kevin Hammel to discover Ms. Guzman's continuous texting and lack of attention to the road. For our Bella, that bus was a rolling torture chamber.

Distracted driving is a national emergency. As a judge, you have before you today an opportunity to send a clear message to Connecticut and the country, that drivers, especially paid commercial drivers, will face the stiffest penalties for endangering everyone on the road.

I have here a petition that I started last Friday. There are 1099 signatures from concerned people around the world asking you to please deny Evelyn Guzman the privilege of accelerated rehabilitation.

Every day she chose to text while driving, she could have killed the children on the bus. She could have killed her own daughter and her grandchildren, who rode her bus as a makeshift daycare center. She showed no regard for fellow drivers or even the unsuspecting person standing at their mailbox or taking a baby for walk.

According to the Trumbull schools transportation department, Guzman's Verizon records showed twenty-seven minutes of texting during a single twenty-eight minute bus route. This may be her first arrest, but it's hardly a first time offense, as the bus videotapes show over and over. This case has been featured on national TV, the Internet, and in print news. I hope to be able to tell the millions of people watching this case that she will stand and face her charges without benefit of accelerated rehabilitation.

April is Autism Awareness month, and I can't think of a better way to voice our support than to protect the children, like my Bella, who can not speak for or protect themselves.

Thank you.

To our dismay, the judge granted Guzman accelerated rehabilitation. He imposed stiff penalties, however. Guzman lost her license to drive any vehicle for two years, can never drive a school bus again, must serve 200 hours in the community, and donate $500 to an autism charity. I gave the State's Attorney the name of a local organization called The Pilot House for her donation.

When the two cases were closed I felt deflated, not jubilant. I had no need for revenge, and it was never my goal to see these two women (whom I had liked) raked over the coals. That said, I wasn't going away quietly (there's a shock). I blogged the cases at every opportunity to keep my friends and the autism family in the loop and to make sure that texting while driving is taken seriously.

And harming a child even more so. The silver lining is that Bella received an outpouring of support from every corner of the autism community, and that was wonderful.

You are the eyes, ears, and voice for my girls and thousands of others with autism. Your kids will be Mia, Bella, and Gianna's peers. They will vote for the laws that protect and care for them, and the taxes that will pay for their services.

I need you. My girls and tens of thousands of kids on their way to becoming adults need you.

Are you ready?

KIM'S GLUTEN-FREE FAMILY RECIPES

Gluten-free Casein-free Macaroni and "Cheese"

1 container Imagine brand Potato Leek Soup
1 bag Daiya brand milk-free/soy-free "cheddar cheese"
1 tsp salt
1 tsp pepper
1 bag gluten-free macaroni (we use Trader's Joe's organic
   brown rice pasta)
GFCF breadcrumbs or crushed potato chips for topping

Boil macaroni in large pasta pot; cook a minute or two less than
the directions suggest
Drain macaroni in sink, leave in colander
In pasta pot mix potato soup, Daiya cheese, salt and pepper, and
cook on low/medium heat until fully blended
Stir macaroni into pot
Pour into greased 9 x 13" pan
Sprinkle with GFCF breadcrumbs or chips
Bake at 350 for 30 minutes
You can divide this recipe into two 8 x 8" pans and freeze one
portion

Gluten-free meatballs
(use organic meats and eggs when budget allows)

1 pound hamburger
½ pound ground pork
½ pound ground veal
2 large eggs
1 cup GF breadcrumbs
Unsweetened coconut milk or water
Salt
Pepper
Onion powder
Fresh minced or jarred minced garlic

Wash your hands and take off any rings

Place the meats into a very large bowl or pot, make a well in the center

Add the eggs, milk or water, garlic, and spices

Squish squish squish with your very clean hands until all ingredients are mixed well

Roll into large or bite sized meatballs

Bake at 375 for about 20 minutes, depending on size, or pan fry in half non-hydrogenated shortening (like Earth Balance or Spectrum brand) and half olive oil until browned and cooked through.

I usually bake them but I fry a "test" meatball to see if the meat is well seasoned.

Easy Stovetop Marinara

1 28-ounce can San Marzano style tomatoes (any brand)
Extra virgin olive oil
3 cloves garlic
Mushrooms
Small can sliced black olives
Kosher salt to taste

Heat oil on medium/low in saucepan
Cook garlic 5 minutes, turn frequently, remove from pan
Brown mushrooms
Add tomatoes, ½ can of water, olives, and salt
Cook 25 minutes, no lid

Hot Fudge

½ cup So Delicious Coconut Milk
1 ½ cups Enjoy Life allergy-free chocolate megachunks
Pinch salt
1 tbsp GFCF margarine (Earth Balance works well)
1 tbsp honey or Karo corn syrup if you can have corn

Bring coconut milk to just under boil in saucepan
Lower heat
Add honey or Karo, chocolate, salt, and margarine
Stir until smooth
Adjust thickness with coconut milk if needed
Eat immediately with large spoon or refrigerate

Sunday Gravy

4 28-ounce cans San Marzano style tomatoes (any brand)
4 cans water
1 large sweet onion
4-6 cloves chopped fresh garlic
Kosher or sea salt
2 bay leaves
Extra virgin olive oil

Put on a Dean Martin CD
Cover bottom of large pot with olive oil 1/8" deep
Saute onion and garlic
Add tomatoes, bay leaves, salt, and water
Bring to boil
Skim foam as it appears (that's acid)
Lower heat, cook 3-4 hours (no lid on pot)
Taste every so often, add salt to taste
Add water if too thick when cooked
If it's acidic to taste, add pinch of sugar

REFERENCES

If you, a family member, or a friend have a loved one diagnosed with autism, this list of resources will provide useful and actionable information on a wide range of topics.

Active Healing: *www.activehealing.org*

Age of Autism: *www.ageofautism.com*

Ask Dr. Sears: *www.askdrsears.com*

Autism diet info: *www.nourishinghope.org*

Autism File Magazine: *www.autismfile.com*

Autism Research Institute: *www.autism.com*

Autism One: *www.autismone.org*

Autism Speaks: *www.autismspeaks.org*

Autism Society of America: *www.autism-society.org*

Center for Autism and Related Disorders: *www.centerforautism.com*

Dr. Andrew Wakefield's book: *www.callous-disregard.com*

Everlon Diamonds (Hey, why not? A girl can dream):
   www.adiamondisforever.com

Generation Rescue: *www.generationrescue.org*

John Robison: *www.johnrobison.com*

Lovaas Center for Applied Behavior Analysis: *www.lovaas.com*

National Autism Association: *www.nationalautismassociation.org*

National Vaccine Information Center: *www.nvic.org*

Pediatric Vaccination Schedules: *www.cdc.gov/vaccines/recs/schedules /child-schedule.htm*

Spectrum Magazine: *www.spectrumpublications.com*

Talk About Curing Autism: *www.talkaboutcuringautism.org*

The Coalition for SafeMinds: *www.safeminds.org*

GLOSSARY OF TERMS

Applied Behavior Analysis (ABA): Applied behavior analysis is the process of systematically applying interventions based upon the principles of learning theory to improve socially significant behaviors to a meaningful degree, and to demonstrate that the interventions employed are responsible for the improvement in behavior (Baer, Wolf & Risley, 1968; Sulzer-Azaroff & Mayer, 1991).

"Socially significant behaviors" include reading, academics, social skills, communication, and adaptive living skills. Adaptive living skills include gross and fine motor skills, eating and food preparation, toileting, dressing, personal self-care, domestic skills, time and punctuality, money and value, home and community orientation, and work skills.

Autism: From the National Autism Association Website: Autism is a bio-neurological developmental disability that generally appears before the age of three. Autism impacts the normal development of the brain in the areas of social interaction, communication skills, and cognitive function. Individuals with autism typically have difficulties in verbal and non-verbal communication, social interactions, and leisure or play activities. Individuals with autism often suffer from numerous physical ailments, which may include: allergies, asthma, epilepsy, digestive disorders, persistent viral infections, feeding disorders, sensory integration dysfunction, sleeping disorders, and more. Autism is diagnosed four times more often in boys than girls. Its prevalence is not affected by race, region, or socio-economic status. Since autism was first diagnosed in the U.S., the occurrence has climbed to an alarming one in 150 people across the country. Autism does not affect life expectancy. Currently there is no cure for autism, though with early intervention and treatment, the diverse symptoms related to autism can be greatly improved.

Bella: Means beautiful in Italian. (Thank goodness our Bella is a beauty. That would have been a tragic irony the child did not need.)

Biomedical Treatment: Autism treatments that include the use of prescription and nonprescription medications, supplements, diet, and other alternative methods to treat the physical manifestations of autism spectrum disorder with the assumption that addressing the physical issues will lead to an improvement in the behavioral and psychological symptoms.

Casein: The protein found in milk.

Crapisode: (From the Urban Dictionary. Really, go look!) An autism-related event involving a child, poop, and typically the walls, carpeting, and often the child him/herself. First used in this context by a mom of three kids with autism who also happens to write. (Guess who?)

Gianna: Female Italian given name, a form of Giovanna meaning "God's grace."

Gluten: The protein found in wheat, oats, and rye.

Mia: Means "mine" in Italian.

Neurodiversity: Neurodiversity is the concept that atypical neurological development is a normal human difference and not what many would call a "brain injury" or disability.

Patterning: A series of movements that mirrors the basics of a baby crawling and creeping.

Stagliano: "They stand out" according to the Babel Fish English to Italian translator. That sounds about right.

BOOK CLUB OR CLASSROOM QUESTIONS

Q) Do you know anyone with autism, adult or child?

Q) What fact(s) did you learn that you didn't know prior to reading this book?

Q) Where do you disagree with the author. Why?

Q) What factors do you think could be causing the increase in autism?

Q) Are you fearful that you might have a child or grandchild with autism in the future?

Q) How do you face adversity in your own life? What coping mechanisms of Kim's did you admire (if any)?

Q) Do you think we should be funding medical treatments and/or seeking a cure for autism, as we do for other illnesses?

Q) Do you think vaccinations play a role in autism? If so, how?

Q) What action can you take to help an affected family after reading this book?

Q) Have you used the term "crapisode" in a conversation yet?